ABOUT THE AUTHOR

Born in 1907, Dr. J. M. Jussawalla graduated from Davidson College of Natural Therapeutics in England and was appointed an assistant to Dr. V. Stanley Davidson of Lindhlar College, U.S.A. On his return to India, he founded the Natural Therapy Clinic in Bombay in 1938. In 1947, Dr. Jussawalla was elected the All India Official Delegate to the Golden Jubilee Congress of the American Naturopathic Association of which he has been a permanent member since then. He was also appointed a member of the Planning Commission on its Health Panel and an adviser to the Government of India on nature cure and served on the Nature Cure Advisory Board of the Government of Gujarat. Dr. Jussawalla is a Director and President in India of the International Federation of the Scientific Research Society for the Prevention of Diseases by Drugless Methods and Fellow of the Naturopathic Forest University where he received his doctorate in Physical Medicine in 1957.

An honorary director and lecturer at the Physiotherapy Centre for the Blind in Bombay, Dr. Jussawalla is also the Vice-President of the All India Nature Cure Federation (Akhil Bharatiya Prakritik Chikitsa Parishad). He is a practising member of the Health Practitioners Association of London, and has been appointed a Special Representative of the International Society of USA Naturopathic Physicians for India.

Dr. Jussawalla is the Vice Chairman of the Vegetarian Society, Bombay, and President of Nature Cure Practitioners Guild (Bombay). He is a member of the governing body of the Central Council for Research in Yoga and Naturopathy, and also of its Scientific and Financial Advisory Committee (Naturopathy). Dr. Jussawalla has authored many books on nature cure, vegetarianism, diet and health.

BY THE SAME AUTHOR

Natural Dietetics

Heal Your Mind, Heal Your Body

The Key to Nature Cure

Vegetarianism

Medical Dietetics

Health For All

Living the Natural Way

Healing from Within

Nature's Materia Medica

INTEGRATED HEALING ARTS

A New Dimension and Revolution in Medicine

DR. J.M. JUSSAWALLA

POPULAR PRAKASHAN
BOMBAY

POPULAR PRAKASHAN PRIVATE LIMITED

35-C, Pandit Madan Mohan Malaviya Marg
Popular Press Bldg., Tardeo, Bombay 400 034

First Published 1988

Second Edition 1993

(4039)

ISBN 81-7154-770-2

Phototypeset by Popular Prakashan Pvt. Ltd., 35-C, Pandit Madan Mohan Malaviya Marg, Tardeo, Bombay 400 034.

Printed in India by Gopsons Papers Pvt. Ltd., A-28, Sector ix, Noida.

Published by Ramdas Bhatkal for Popular Prakashan Pvt. Ltd., 35-C, Pandit Madan Mohan Malaviya Marg, Tardeo, Bombay 400 034.

Dedicated to the
Universal School of Medicine

The Hippocratic Oath

I SWEAR by Apollo, the physician; Asclepius, Hygieia, and Panacea; invoking all the gods and goddesses to be my witnesses, that I will fulfil this Oath and this written covenant to the best of my powers and judgement. I will look upon him who shall have taught me this art even as on mine own parents; I will share with him my substance, and supply his necessities if he be in need. I will regard his offspring even as my own brethren, and will teach them this art, if they desire to learn it without fee or covenant.

I WILL IMPART it by precept, by lecture and by all other manner of teaching, not only to my own sons but also to the sons of him who has taught me, and to the disciples bound by covenant and oath according to the law of the physicians, and to none other.

THE REGIMEN I adopt shall be for the benefit of the patients to the best of my power and judgement; it shall not be for their injury or for any wrongful purpose. I will not give a deadly drug to any one, though it be asked of me, nor will I lead the way in such counsel; and likewise I will not give a woman a pessary to procure abortion. But I will keep my life and my art in purity and holiness. I will not use the knife, not even, verily, on sufferers from stone, but I will give reference to such as are craftsmen therein.

WHATSOEVER HOUSE I enter, I will enter for the benefit of the sick, refraining from all voluntary wrong-doing and corruption, especially seduction of male or female, bonded or free.

WHATSOEVER THINGS I see or hear concerning the life of men, in my attendance on the sick or even apart from my attendance, which ought not to be blabbed abroad, I will keep silence on them, counting such things to be as religious secrets.

IF I FULFIL THIS oath and confound it not, be it mine to enjoy life and art alike, with good repute among all men for all time to come; but the contrary befall me if I transgress and violate my oath.

Introduction

Various systems of medicine and therapy are practised in the world of healing : medical, surgical, ayurveda, homoeopathy, nature cure, biochemic remedies, other universal healing methods and systems. As a rule the physician practises according to the doctrine prevailing in the particular school of thought in which he is trained. Some controversy usually arises amongst the practitioners of different systems and therapies as their premises for thinking are based on their training in a particular school of medicine.

We view with alarm the tremendous increase in degenerative diseases and failing health.

Progress in any scientific endeavour is but the investigation and improvement of the respective technique and the development of new and better application. The healing art is no exception.

No science, however variable, can be allowed to stagnate in its doctrine and refuse to move and adapt itself to changing circumstances of the world.

The philosophy of change and the mutability of scientific dicta justify the birth of yet another Institute for a close inquiry into the rights and merits of apparent theories on the most vital aspects of life, viz. Health and Longevity.

In the condition of this universe the greatest need of the hour in this sphere, is a wide diffusion of enlightenment regarding the ways to maintain and improve health and to avoid sickess. What we need today is a Universal Health Institute - an Institute of Integrated Healing Arts and Paramedical Science on Health and Disease where different systems of medicine and therapies are practised on Preventive and Curative Lines. (The Holistic approach into the whole system of medicine.)

The aim of the Institute representing different systems of medicine and various therapies is to work in harmony without a shadow of misunderstanding, jealousy or intolerance; laying aside bigotry and narrowness - a catholic approach; exemplifying true eclecticism avoiding, at the same time, such methods which are treacherous and destructive to health and life.

The ancient sages, rishis and healers taught and practised the art of healing over thousands of years ago, but the laws and methods were lost and buried with other wisdom of the ancients and modern until re-discovered and revered by the healers of Rational Medicine.

The need of the moment is for co-ordination of various methods and therapies for co-operation between those on different lines so that patients may find the treatment suited to their case without undue experiment and delay.

J. M. JUSSAWALLA

Contents

PART III

PART IV

Part I

"There is no treasure like knowledge
and knowledge is nothing but finding
unity in the midst of diversity."

1. Health for All

Health is the most important special
index of the quality of life.

The greatest need of the hour is how to attain and maintain health and prevent disease, inspite of the odds facing us in the exacting artificial demands and tensions of the modern civilized life. In the industrial age in which we are living, it is difficult to evade a stereotyped pattern of life which overlooks the importance of health acquisitiveness though we know the indispensable fact that neglect of the faculty of our being brings in its trail ill-health, disease and suffering.

Health is indisputably the most valued of all possessions a person aspires for. Although it may be neglected unconsciously, it is an inescapable fact that wealth without health or happiness without health is incomplete. Hence the emphasis primarily on health even at national levels.

The state of health implies much more than freedom from disease, and good health may be defined as the attainment and maintenance of the highest state of mental and bodily vigour.

A healthy body is attested by its functions being carried out without discomfort, by the capacity for exertion appropriate to the age of the individual and without undue fatigue, and by its possessing such reserves of energy as are adequate to the ordinary emergencies of everyday life. Thus in the healthy man or woman food is digested, blood sent circulating throughout the body, the lungs aerated without any of its myriad functions obtruding itself on the consciousness. Similarly, a healthy mind is adequate to such work as would reasonably be expected of it.

This is about "adequate" functioning of the body, a thing apart from "prime" functioning. It should be possible to live with gusto: to have an appetite for work and play which is equally keen, a generous fountain of energy should surge up within us and the exercise of brain or muscle should be in the highest degree pleasurable. This degree of health is seen often enough in young people, but though it is sometimes enjoyed by their elders it is not nearly so common as it might be. It is not sought after by very many, because its possibility is doubted, others are too indolent to bother about it, while some find too many obstacles in the way.

People in general give very little attention to health until it is destroyed. Then they call in a doctor thinking their responsibility has ended; the idea being that health and disease are largely matters of chance and that the responsibility rests with the doctor. This is wrong thinking.

No improvement in the health care system can be efficacious unless the individual assumes responsibility for his own well-being. There are substantial latent gains in health care education because those who accept responsibility for self-care are healthier than those who are dependent on others to detect their ill health. For the old adage "prevention is better than cure" to fructify, every person would have to study the art of right living.

There are doubtless many factors and reasons such as pollution, adulteration of food, facing the stress and strain of modern life which give rise to modern health problems. But these may be lessened by corrective commercial action and by individual effort and care. Other methods of healthy living lie in consciously-cultivated habits, which are under individual control.

Fight Against Micro-organisms

Micro-organisms are responsible for one-third of the world's diseases. While many of the methods of combating these may be allocated to the sanitary authorities, much can be done by individual action. The first step being to understand the nature of such organisms and of the ways in which they should be eliminated.

A high degree of personal cleanliness as well as that of the home should be maintained, the destruction of flies and other insect carriers of disease; vigilant protection of food should be carried out; food which is possibly infected should be sterilised, and antiseptics and disinfectants should be intelligently used whenever and wherever necessary. The Mosaic law of washing the hands before taking food is no mere ceremonial, and not only in feeding but while handling food the hands should be clean.

There are two sources of bacterial poisoning which are responsible for a large number of not only minor maladies and generally low conditions of health, but also of serious disease; these sources are the mouth and the bowel.

Food and Digestion

Related to these subjects, both as cause and effect, are those concerning food and digestion. Because of the fact that much of the food required is exported, that such a large proportion of the population lives in towns, where fresh foodstuffs are difficult of access and that there is so much refinement leading to overcooking and use of excessive spices in the preparation of food, that it has become habitual for us to take improper food. There is too little fresh food, and especially fresh fruit, vegetables and dairy produce in the diet of many households.

In too many instances ill-health is due to insufficiency of food. This comes about due to an unskillful choice of food, and unhealthy and unattractive methods of cooking. There are many cheap foods which are very nutritious and which skill in cookery may make as appetising as more expensive foods. A widespread knowledge of food values and nutritional preparation would prove invaluable in improving the health of the masses.

A common mistake among well-to-do people is to take an excess of food. Good cooking helps the digestion of food enormously, but it may easily tempt one to eat in excess; and when this becomes habitual it brings serious trouble in its wake. Good and balanced nutrition is the surest safeguard against most of the preventible diseases.

Fresh Air and Sunshine

In some quarters there is still a prejudice against the open bedroom window; sinister properties are attributed to the night air. But nothing could be farther from the truth, as it has been proved experimentally that the night air is freer from suspended impurities than the air during the day. Moreover, it has been demonstrated that the chief virtue of fresh air is the stimulation imparted by its circulation about our bodies, and that one feels better in purer air which is still than in stale air which is circulating freely. Few people seem to realize how many hours they spend in a bedroom and how unwholesome it must be to have the circulation of air prevented by closed windows. Draughts have a terror for many, but a free current of air over the bedclothes cannot do any harm, besides the wider the window is open the less the draught.

It ought to be commonly known that the healthy rays of the sun do not make their way through windows made of ordinary glass. The importance of the violet rays is a comparatively recent discovery, but the lack of exposure to them coupled with bad ventilation in a room and not enough exercise undoubtedly explains the discounted state of health of the sedentary worker and of the housewife who rarely goes beyond her doorstep.

Importance of Exercise

To most people games are more interesting than mere walking and they do afford better exercise; but it should not be forgotten that before taking up a strenuous game, a sedentary worker should make himself first of all fit by a course of graduated gymnastics or easier kinds of outdoor exercise. Active men or women who find that there is no time for games should supplement outdoor walking by exercising in their rooms for a few minutes each day, the exercises chosen being such that bring as many muscles as possible into play and which move the joints as freely as possible.

For others the prescription may be different; they may require more rest, and in particular a longer time in bed, about seven or eight hours as a rule. In bed the muscles of the body are allowed to relax properly, for it always requires some muscular effort to maintain even a sitting posture; the heart rate reduces and the heart gets more rest, and the brain and other portions of the nervous system get time for rest. To ensure a proper night's rest, strenuous mental work should not be engaged in just before bedtime.

It is often said that the best rest is a change of occupation, and there is a considerable amount of truth in this. Turning to a fresh subject of thought or a different kind of manual occupation tends to prevent staleness and fatigue, and a larger volume of work may be achieved in this way. Hence the health value of an absorbing hobby for the leisure hours. But discretion must be shown in pursuing such a plan in moderation, or the cumulative effect of a variety of occupations may drain one's reserves of energy unduly.

The main clauses of the charter of health have now been considered, and if they are understood and followed there need be no fussy pre-occupation about the functioning of the body. In many respects the body can be likened to a machine. Its mechanism is intricate and delicate but it differs from an ordinary machine in its inherent powers of adjustment and control, in its powers of resistance to cause of disease and its power of repair. The essential components of the body are living cells, each of which will put up a fight for life and comfort.

A sane balanced method of living affords this commonwealth of body cells the best opportunity to fulfil their destiny. A succession of fads in the matter of diet and indiscriminate resort to drugs of one kind or another only impedes and confuses the natural immune system. If the body gets the right kind of food and a sufficiency of oxygen, and is kept free from waste products by the regular action of the excretory organs of the body, it is best left alone. In exceptional circumstances a system of diet or the action of a drug may become necessary.

Health of the Mind

Many people go through their lives dogged by the haunting fear of this or that disease. Fear has a depressing influence on the body, and there are curious instances of individuals succumbing to the very disease which they dread-'That which I feared has come upon me.'

The notion of hygiene of the body is familiar to most, but few people are so alive to the necessity of the hygiene of the mind. The kind of ideas that form the content of the mind is not a matter of indifference to the health of either mind or body. Just as the body must be supplied with wholesome food and be purged from deleterious substances, so must the mind be supplied with sane, healthy ideas and be cleared of such as are the opposite.

Thinking is not confined to the brain. The whole body participates in it. The mind, especially the emotions are among the most powerful influences which affect the body. Joy, sorrow, anger, fear and other emotional states may exalt or depress bodily functions as quickly and as powerfully as the most potent drugs or the most active physical agents. The relation between the body and mind is so intimate that if either gets out of order the whole system suffers.

There are various methods propounded for the study of the knowledge of oneself and of the mind in relation to health, such as Metaphysical Science, Psychology, Yoga, Philosophy, Theosophy, Occultism, Christian Science, Vegetarianism, Hypnotism, Astrology, faith, prayer and meditation, spiritual healing, etc. Call it by any name, health is the result of living in accordance with the laws that operate in the mind, emotions and sense impressions; such knowledge helps one to reveal one's truest worth. The idea that our own thoughts play a decisive role in health and illness presents us with an enormous responsibility, one which we previously delegated entirely to physicians.

Sickness in ancient times, was largely due to ignorance of the physical laws governing health. Hippocrates, popularly known as "The Moses of medicine," in his time, led the physician from the Egyptian darkness of magic and superstition into the pronounced law of rational therapy.

In the modern world, sickness is more often the result of ignorance of the laws governing the mental, emotional and spiritual forces operating in people's lives. In our efforts to conquer externals we have failed to meet the challenge of the internal existence. Prevention or the positive building of health and mental hygiene should be the aim and object of the Healing Arts, as positive health is the only true prophylactic or means of immunity against disease.

2. Medicine

Medicine in the nineteenth century was concerned chiefly with the study of disease. The discovery of germs, what Pasteur called "the kingdom of the infinitely small," opened the doors of a new world. Every physician was eager to enter and possess it. Thus through bacteriology, man was master of the germs of disease, and became the most prominent figure on the stage. He told his admiring colleagues that this or that infirmity was due to this or that bacillus, and that if the germ could be destroyed the malady would disappear from the earth. The very highest hopes were formed; the most extravagant ideals were put forth as serious contributions to scientific progress.

It would be wrong and stupid to deny that great benefits have been obtained from this attack on the germs of disease. We owe much of our safety and fitness to bacteriology. It has given us purer water, cleaner and more wholesome food and freedom from many infections. Nor are its services in these directions by any means exhausted. It has given us also a new insight into the spread of disease and into the subtle and wonderful methods by which nature defends herself against attacks.

But most medical men of our day seem to think that their task is to prescribe drugs or injections which they learn so assiduously in the orthodox medical schools and colleges of the Western system and which they are taught to believe to be the only way to relieve the suffering of the sick. There ends their duty to the suffering humanity. The mental make-up of the patient and the environment in which he lives are almost completely overlooked or ignored. The chemists and druggists generally guide the prescriptions that will be written by medical practitioners. It seldom occurs to them that, they being the arbiters of people's health, it is incumbent on them to disseminate true health knowledge to their patients so that they may be able to raise the standards of their health. Preventing the onset of disease is as important as to get it cured, specially when we can reasonably presume that it is common knowledge to physicians that a lower standard of health coupled with a sheer neglect of mental hygiene methods are mainly responsible for reducing the resistance of the body to disease.

Scientists are busy in their own way to check the spread of disease by new discoveries of so-called wonder drugs, antibiotics, vaccines, sera, and so on. They have, no doubt, been able to arrest the progress of certain diseases by the conjoint application of their experimental remedial agents along with hygienic methods. But are these remedies, changing as they are from time to time, reliable and free from all harmful after-effects on the human system? The answer is to be found in the millions of suffering men, women and children, seeking the aid of any and every other system of medicine, after either having failed to get redress or relief of their sufferings in the hands of the so-called practitioners of the scientific western system of medicine, or because it is beyond their means to avail of them. Many honest, conscientious, highly qualified and experienced medical professors of the western system have denounced, in unequivocal terms, the practice of the medical science in its present form and the claims made by it.

Quite a few eminent physicians have mentioned that the art of healing has gone astray:

"Up-to-date orthodox medical researchers have been working either in cul-de-sacs or in circles constantly receding further from the centre. They have been obsessed with microbes or viruses and have been responsible for the idea that disease may be conquered by injecting man's long-suffering body with sera, vaccines, toxins or chemicals.Their work has a pernicious effect upon medical education so that the student is encouraged to lean upon laboratory findings and to disregard experience and observation; their work has encouraged specialization just as if the human body were divisible into a large number of more or less water-tight compartments and furthermore, the manufacturing chemists are inundating medical men and the general public with all kinds of preparations founded upon what they call ' medical science'."

Undoubtedly, the invention of some wonder drugs, the facilities extended by modern hospitals for indoor and emergency cases, and with the jet-age service and cure for critically-ill patients, have reduced the rate of mortality as the progressive physician prolongs life by any means in his power on the assumption that hope lingers until actual death. Besides, from the point of view of modern civilized life-style, especially the urban life-style, the treatment of illness and disease has become much popular resulting in medical epidemic and the universality of the medical system.

3. Surgery

The progress and triumph of modern surgery has been brought about through the evolution of three interrelated factors :

(i) Anesthetics : These marvellous drugs are perhaps the most obvious blessings in the history of medicine, permitting, as they do, the painless performance of the most extensive and prolonged operations.

(ii) Manual skill : The safety of operative procedure, even today, is largely dependent upon the manual dexterity and especially the expeditiousness of the surgeon. Only by painstaking experience in actual practice can such technical perfection be attained.

(iii) Asepsis : Neither absence of pain, nor skill in the operator, would avail much unless the great principle of cleanliness, or asepsis, to give it its scientific designation, were applied vigorously in every surgical procedure.

Of all the new surgical life-saving techniques, the bypass surgery and the most medically invasive - and perhaps, the most promising, is the transplants of human organs. The most important and baffling difficulty in the way of successful transplants is immunological rejection, the individual body's destructive reaction to tissue other than its own. This reaction usually rejects transplanted organs and so the method in such cases tends to become a short-term affair unless some other means to slow down the rejection process are adopted.

Alternative health system has a great respect for the art of surgery when practised in a constructive manner. It appreciates the facts, as mentioned above, that there are conditions in which surgery is necessary and is a boon in an emergency, but when resorted to unnecessarily, it would be considered a most unethical practice on the part of the surgeon. Nobody, therefore, would declaim against the true science of surgery, which as a leading medical man declared: "The medical facts of today are fallacies of tomorrow; when conditions and circumstances demand surgical intervention and assistance, there is no substitute."

4. Nature Cure

The basis of Natural Healing is character.

As a science, bacteriology has not given us that complete dominance over disease which many expected, and so, little by little, the other side of the problem, the human body, has regained attention. The medicine of the twentieth century is chiefly concerned with the study of health and hence the term Rational Medicine is no longer new. Physicians are moving in sympathy with those rational and physiological means, which are often slow to show immediate results, but which act with a certainty and permanency that cannot be ascribed to other agents, which if active at all, are only active as toxic agents. Rational medicine does not seek to cure disease by a system of antidoting one poison by another, or by neutralising the effects of one morbid action by artificially creating another of an opposite kind.

Rational medicine seeks first to find and remove the cause of disease, and then to aid the body in its efforts to combat disease by means of all natural and rational remedies, such as light, water, air, heat, exercise, diet and other physiological measures.

Nature cure, naturopathy, the natural methods, the new science of healing, healing from within, are different names for the same method. It is built upon the dictum of Hippocrates, who declared "Nature Cures; not the physicians". He was one of the great minds to base the practice of medicine upon principles of inductive philosophy and to direct special attention to the natural history of disease.

Historically, eclectic or progressive naturopathy can trace its origin back to Hippocrates, the father of medicine, in whose writings are found that great reliance was placed upon the 'vis medicatrix naturea' -- the healing power of nature, and the idea that 'nature heals, the physician assists.'

At no time did Hippocrates or his contemporaries teach or instruct that one particular method or system of healing was sufficient to maintain or restore the health of man -- "use every available means necessary for the particular case". Hippocrates taught "the first aim in the practice of the healing art is how to make the patient well and, if the patient can be made well in more than one way, choose the least troublesome."

The close relationship existing between the three basic branches of the healing arts cannot be ignored. The triad of healing through nutrition, through medication and through the hand, makes them inseparable and tremendously strong in all of their phases; they are as inseparable as are the mind and body.

According to the naturopathic concept of diseases, their causes,diagnosis, treatment and prevention, as well as the composition, structure and function of the human organism may be classified into three categories: the psychological, the physiological, and the chemical. The advanced naturopathic physician does not regard naturopathy as a rigid system in the dogmatic sense. Naturopathy is primarily and fundamentally drugless and 'bloodless' yet in its broader aspects it does admit the use of both natural medicine and surgery when their use is constructive. The individual modalities and techniques employed in nature cure vary with the degree of intelligence, training and clinical experience of its practitioner. Besides, there is constant change in the methods of healing. Progress in any scientific endeavour is but the investigation and improvement of the respective techniques and the development of new and better application. The healing art is no exception, and progress is made in all of its branches. Various techniques and systems have made enough progress within the last century and a half to warrant their utilization extensively. Any and every healing method which is constructive, and not repressive, and which conforms in every respect to the philosophy of the science should be conjointly used if necessary to get the best results for the patient.

Life has become complicated and is becoming increasingly so. Today, man, having departed from the simplicity of Nature, has entered into myriad complications which have multiplied his many difficulties. Therefore, progressive doctors and scientists are again calling for a return to the art of sensible living in a bid to restore a sense of harmony to human life.

5. Ayurveda

It is said that the ancient rishis -- those powerful sages -- brought the knowledge of medicine and passed down to others who started the University of Taxila, perhaps the most important centre of learning in ancient India. One of the pupils wrote the treatise which formed the basis of the great textbook, the *Charaka Samhita* which remains central to Ayurveda training to this day.

Ayurveda, an indigenous system of medicine, is the ancient science of life. It uses herbs extensively for various cures. Ayurveda covers the animal and the vegetable kingdom. Like the human beings, the vegetable world is also subject to *vata* (the wind), *paitta* (the bile) and *kapha* (the phlegm) disorders and has to be treated accordingly. But the main subject of treatment is man. His contact with unpleasantness is termed 'disease.'

Tridosha vada (psycho-physio pathology) of the living organism as one compact whole, special diet, herbal decoction, fomentation and massage, enema in its various forms are special features of Ayurveda which could be stated as a judicious combination of the principles of nature cure as well. It alters the body's chemistry in a way that relieves the symptoms.

Says Charaka, "Nothing exists in the world of thought or experience that cannot be used as medicine". Knowledge of medicinal herbs and drugs was based on popular experience and was mostly empirically accumulated and spread. But alchemy was not without its influence on the further development of medicaments, although many errors were made, but now we can get a clear picture from the various pharmacopias which were later revised and scientifically proved.

Like the Chinese acupuncture, the Chinese systematic breathing exercises, (the latter considered as a more dynamic system of body movements than the Indian system of yoga), there is also a vast heritage of Chinese medicinal herbs having great medicinal value in the art of healing.

For instance, the *Ginseng root* is an important medicinal herb. It is a tonic, an excellent means of tonification for the central nervous system and a first class regulator of high blood pressure. It is also effective in cases of diabetes. It is said to contain phosphorus, potassium, calcium, magnesium, sodium, iron, aluminium, silicon, barium, strontium, manganese, titonium, glucose and volatile oil. It is used for vigour and vitality. This root is similar to the human body; the two tips of the root are like legs and the two upper continuations of the root are like arms, this was why this wonderful rare plant became known and celebrated as the 'herb of eternal life' as well as the 'elixir.' Although modern medicine has found that it does not confer eternal life, Ginseng is so popular throughout the world that it is also called 'a wonder of the world.'

Ayur means life and *veda* means science and a major portion of ayurveda, the science of life, deals with the rules of daily routine, normal health, hygiene, and seasonal regulations, in which diet is also included.

The traditional art of healing also discriminates between medicaments of cold and warm nature. In ancient times it was thought that illnesses of a 'warm' nature should be cured by 'cold' medicaments, and vice versa. In addition, medicaments were also divided according to their taste -- bitter, sour, salty, and sharp ones being considered suitable for the curing of different ailments. "A bitter taste has a 'hard', 'strong' character and affects the heart; a sour taste, which influences the liver, has a 'composing' character; a sweet taste has mild qualities and affects the functioning of the spleen; the 'delicate' nature of a salty taste affects the kidney and the urinary bladder; sharp, 'dispersing' taste affects the lungs."

This differentiation between the qualities of various tastes and their association with specific illnesses represents a notable discovery, already some thousands of years old, on the part of the ancient science of life.

The connection between the heart and bitterness of taste may be roughly explained as follows: one of the chief symptoms of disorders of the biliary system is that the secretion of bile becomes congested and, as a result, congeals. Because of this difficulty in emptying the gall bladder some bile penetrates the blood system, and its bitter taste is felt by the tongue and the papillae of the mouth. The patient has thus a continual bitter taste in his mouth; whatever he eats and drinks also tastes bitter. This irritation of the biliary duct exerts a reflex effect on the vessels of the heart and causes attacks similar to angina pectoris. Nevertheless, the heart itself is absolutely sound, for this is essentially a case of visceral reflexes between it and the biliary system. Consequently, whenever a patient complains of attacks similar to angina pectoris and at the same time has a bitter taste in his mouth, then the chances are that the trouble lies with the gall bladder and not the heart.

The connection between a sour taste and the liver can be explained by the fact that chronic diseases of the liver are usually accompanied by inflammation of the mucous membrane of the stomach and an excess production of acid. It is mainly the biliary capillaries inside the liver which are affected, and the disease is transmitted to the stomach. The disordered state of the biliary capillaries is due to chronic dysfunction of the hepatic cells of which their walls are formed. This category of patients always have a sour taste in the mouth, indicating a disorder of the liver.

The spleen and the pancreas can be regarded as belonging to one unified system, though the ancient Chinese did not know of the pancreas as such. They were justified in regardng the two as one unit inasmuch as the symptomatology of the points on the spleen meridian includes the entire functional sphere of the pancreas as well. Western books on acupuncture often also describe this meridian as the spleen-pancreas meridian. We also know that the pancreas is, in addition, one of the main organs controlling sugar content in the body, and the direct effect of sweet food (carbohydrates) on this system is well known.

Another commonly known fact is that sufferers from kidney diseases should not eat strongly salted food. The susceptibility of such people to edema is closely bound with the quantity of sodium and chlorine in the body and its control.

Many of these opinions which had been formed purely empirically have been confirmed by modern findings.

If a modern herbalist were to say "We are specialists in curing the incurable, it sounds somewhat dramatic forgetting there are no incurable diseases, only patients. Take any disease curable or incurable in any field of medicine, much depends on the vital force of the patient, in what stage the disease is, and how much damage has been done by the time the patient comes to the healer."

6. Homoeopathy

Homoeopathy is an art based upon science and it satisfies all the rules of inductive logic. The first and primary rule of Homoeopathy is "treat likes with likes"; select the medicinal agent in any given case of disease, that has produced in healthy human beings manifestations most similar to those present in the diseased individual. The art of homoeopathy demands the proper application of this main rule of the science.

Diseases are characterised by deviations from the normal routine of healthy life. These are called symptoms, and each case of disease is a complex of symptoms. By symptoms is meant here not only phenomena of disease which are subjective, such as pain, but also those that are objective, such as temperature, heat, murmurs and other signs.

Further, when drugs are administered to healthy persons they produce drug - related diseases characterised by distinctive symptoms, so that these conditions also form symptom pictures or symptom complexes.

The essential principle of homoeopathy is that the drug most likely to cure or relieve any case of disease is the drug that would in healthy people produce the symptoms of the disease being treated. In other words, *similus similibus curanter* meaning let likes be treated with likes.

Any symptomatic measure to suppress all outward signs of sickness lurking inside the body reappear in full force with homoeopathic high-potency medication just as with nature cure. When patients are put on a therapeutic fast the manifestation known as 'healing crises' which is Nature's method of getting rid of the poison as well as the suppressed symptoms is mistaken for 'disease crisis.' This is where the difficulty arises because patients switch over to other methods to tide over the so-called 'crisis' in order to get immediate relief by suppressing it, but this does not lead to a cure.

Dr. Hahnemann after experimentation arrived at the conclusion: "It is only the power to make sick that drugs can cure sickness and that a medicine can only cure such morbid condition as it can produce, when tested on healthy persons." Here, the rule is to treat the patient, not the disease.

7. Unani

Another school of medicine called Unani, which was like Ayurveda very popular under the royal patronage of the rulers, asserts that there are four fluids in the human body, namely, red blood, black blood, yellow bile, and white lymph. As in Ayurveda *tridesha* and in other medical sciences, generally speaking, there are three basic types of constitution which, however, may not be found so sharply demarcated.

1) The lymphatic constitution inclines towards gland troubles, scrofula, tuberculosis, skin diseases.

2) The acid type contracts rheumatism, gout, diabetes, artherosclerosis, cardiac affectation, and circulatory disorders, etc.

3) The neuropathic constitution is inclined to all nervous troubles and diseases of the nerves, etc.

Disease, according to the Hippocratic doctrine, was due to the derangement of the 'four humours' or bodily fluids; these were blood, phlegm, black bile, and yellow bile. When these humours were not in proper proportion or arrangement, sickness invariably followed, and if they could be coaxed into a more proportionate relationship a cure could be effected.

The followers of the system known as Hakim, maintain that abnormal and subnormal conditions in these fluids cause disease, and to keep these in normal condition they administer drugs, metals, syrups, jams called *kushtas* (oxides), etc.

8. Biochemistry

Biochemistry or the biochemic treatment of disease is the chemistry of life. It is a system of medicine built upon the biological cycle, that is the branch of science relating to the needs and processes of living organisms (cellular pathology).

An analysis of the blood shows it to contain organic and inorganic matter. The organic constituents are sugar, fats and aluminium substances. The inorganic constituents are water and certain minerals, commonly called cell-salts. The cell-salts are the vital portion of the body and are absolutely essential to their integrity of structure and functional activity.

The theory of Biochemistry is based upon the fact that all the substances necessary to heal, restore and overcome diseased conditions are normally found within the organism itself, and that the structure and vitality of the human body is dependent upon certain necessary quantitites and proper supply of its organic and inorganic constituents. In short Biochemistry is a system of medicine in which health is restored by supplying the deficient cell-salts to the body.

These remedies are quite harmless and if judiciously administered they aid Nature in her efforts to cure by supplying her own remedies work very well; that is why these methods are considered at times as 'home-remedies.'

Biochemistry does not oppose the simultaneous use of other accepted forms of medication against the germ and bacillus, but while such treatment is being carried out, Biochemistry actually goes to the basic cause of the trouble. It supplies to the affected cells, the inorganic organisms of a breeding place, and restores the tissues to a healthy, normal condition.

The twelve tissue salts by their mode of action and therapeutic use represent to some extent the practical basis on which the salts are supplied to the human body. The principles of Biochemic therapy are usually formulated according to the method of Dr. Schussler.

Part II

''Never utter these words
'I do not know this - therefore it is false.'
One must study to know,
know to understand, understand to judge.''

9. The Ancient Cultural Heritage

Old Wine in a New Bottle

What distinguished the medicine of the past is not that its practitioners were well equipped with an amount of antibiotics but they were furnished with a comprehensive and unprecedented understanding of what the healthy body is, how it survives and protects itself. Besides, inspite of varieties of names, the principle behind all these is one of existing nature to do the health restoring work in our own way thereby helping the suffering humanity.

The ancient sages and rishis were furnished with the healing power of nature. They tried to mobilize the natural resources of body and mind in treating patients being acquainted with certain secrets of nature.

Yoga

A practical system of physical, mental and spiritual culture - a way of life and not to be taken as mere physical exercises.

The scientific aspect of the Yoga Science is an Indian heritage received right from Upanishads to the great sage Patanjali. It is so neatly framed that it constitutes an overall effect on the human body and mind. All the pros and cons of the body-mind complex are taken into consideration and various varieties of processes are included in Yoga Science. Dr. Swami Gitanadaji of Pondicherry, a scientist, scholar and a yogi, is highly respected authority on classical Yoga Therapy and Yogic Research. He is an advisor and Guru to several Yoga Centres in India and throughout the world which are operated by his direct disciples.

Hypnosis

It is the power of thought, subconsciously working in a positive way which the mind has come to use when it needs outside help. Hypnosis, therefore, taps the subconscious mind. It is known as 'Mind-Suggestion for psychological trouble.' Suggestion is the subconscious realisation of an idea. The essential characteristic of hypnotic state is the subject's power over his own organism. Hypnosis as a medical reality is a means of therapy and an instrument which can be used as a powerful anesthetic or as non-toxic tranquilizer.

Auto-Suggestion

Auto-Suggestion is self Hypnosis. The most significant phenomena of Auto-Suggestion occur in the domain of the subconscious (Unconscious). The unconscious Auto-Suggestion is responsible for many of our troubles moral and physical. Auto-Suggestion must be concrete or specific, possible and constructive with deep concentration and deep prayer. As the suggestion works on the subconscious mind it is most receptive before going to sleep e.g. 'day by day in every way I am getting better and better.'

Natural Healers

In general most people possess latent healing powers. To possess healing hands is a sure indication that the gift exists but must be latent and needs to be developed. It is a gift of God given to Healers for the benefit of suffering humanity.

Psychic Healing

Man's medical tool is his hands. It is perhaps the oldest of remedies. Each one of us possesses a reservoir of physical and etheric energy and when this is depleted there is lassitude and weakness, laying of hands as in psychic healing by which energy flows from a healer to the patient.

Prayer

There is no greater power for inward protection and divine consciousness than deep prayer and meditation. In meditation you listen to God whereas in prayer you talk to God.

Faith Healing

Faith Healing is an effective mental approach to reality. Prayer and Faith work harmoniously; both are necessary for achievement.

Spiritual Healing - Divine Science

Spiritual Healing is an age old art. In spirit Healing the healer does not heal, he is only an instrument through which it may take place as the healing force emanates from the spirit (departed soul). The human instrument is a channel invoking the aid of the spirit and the vital part the healer plays. The healers can act only as receivers of the healing forces which have been transmitted to the patients and that no human act can produce the healing result. Spiritual Healers are in a position to tap the divine energy within them; that is why it is called Divine Healing.

There are more things in Heaven and Earth than are thought of in the philosophy of the art and science of medicines.

Teletherapy

Tele means distant. Pathy means disease. Teletherapy is a method of curing or healing at a distance without personal presence by using photographs, signatures, etc.

Cosmic rays are radiated to the photographs reaching to the patient penetrating his Aura, which is considered the place of disease.

The Aura is a radiation that is seen to surround the physical body. It possesses different colours, indicates the harmony and disharmony state of body and mind, the state of personal health etc., according to the purity of colour. The colours of the various gem stones are used (with reference to the astrological birth chart of the patient) to supply the colour deficiency in the aura of the patient and restore health.

Astro Medicine

Astro Medicine or Medical Astrology is the science and art of obtaining scientific knowledge regarding diseases and helps to understand the type of the constitution and mental behaviour of the patient. The combination of the science of astrological and medical health can become one of the best methods in the health field. It is the study of man's response to planetary stimuli and the latent tendencies are foreshown. Astrology is too vast a science and an art to be rightly grasped mathematically and philosophically except by those of profound understanding as it is said that intuitive wisdom is essential for right interpretation of the chart. Astrology with the science of occultation is the most valuable asset to a healer from a diagnostic point of view.

The Water of Life

Our body distils the most wonderful medicine and provides the most perfect serums and antibodies.

Human Urine in medical parlance is known as Elixir or Water of Life. Urine Therapy is not new. It was used by the ancient people to preserve their health. A domestic remedy for curing various physical troubles. Among gypsies the health giving properties have been known for centuries. Dr. John W. Armstrong who introduced his therapy in the West writes "The Urine Therapy is a Nature Cure in the most liberal sense of the word and to employ measures which are contrary to the nature at the same time, would not only be quite illogical but even dangerous." In fact such a method of treatment on preventive lines under nature cure has not been generally included because of want of knowledge and study in the field. Urine Therapy as a remedy requires much study and research so that it can be prescribed in lieu of other measures when they fail.

Meditation

Success in any programme of meditation depends upon concentration and relaxation. Constant practise of concentration enables one to give entire attention on prayer. Under circumstances of stress, even leading to "fight" or "fright", the way of stopping the process is "relaxation".

It will be useful to furnish a brief exposition of some of the techniques of the healing art for the promotion of health, prevention and cure of disease.

These are not platitudes, but facts.

10. Acupuncture

Acupuncture, also known as needling, is a form of a surgical procedure devised in China. It is the insertion of fine steel, silver or gold needles into selected areas of the skin as a remedy for disease.

Insertion of the needle in different ways results in weak or strong stimuli being administered to the body.

Rules of acupuncture are numerous and these laws must be observed to reach each medium having a chronological position which it always occupies as the life-force flows through the body.

The meridian of an organ is composed of all points in the body by which the organ in question is primarily affected.

The energy circulating through the entire body regulates the circulation of the blood, ingestion and the auto-protection of the organism. It also flows along the meridian. If it is hindered from circulating or blocked as the result of some external or endogenous circumstances an abnormal surplus or lack of energy results.

If the functioning of an organ begins to fail, it must be strengthened; on the other hand, in the event of hyperfunction the excess of ''energy' must, as it were, be drawn off. Thus tonification and sedation imply that harmony can be restored through the application of stimulating or subduing treatment at the relevant points on the body. In other words, tonification represents ''strong, persistent stimulation,'' whereas sedation means a weak, calming influence.

Since it is supposed to relieve internal congestion and to restore the equilibrium of the bodily functions, acupuncture has been used for a vast variety of diseases and especially for the treatment of arthritis, headache, convulsions, lethargy, colic, etc.

Acute neuralgia or sciatica is treated successfully with acupuncture. In obstinate sciatica it is often very successful. The needles are pushed into the sciatic nerve and left there for 20 to 30 minutes. The insertion causes very little pain.

Another use of acupuncture is in the treatment of aneurysm. Here needles are pushed into the aneurysmal sac or dilated part of the artery. They are made to extend far enough to reach the inner lining of the sac, which they scratch as they are moved about by the blood flow. This leads to the deposit of thrombus, or clot on the vessel lining, and this may go on till the sac is filled with clot and obliterated.

Acupuncture at times plays an important role in surgery not as general anaesthetic agent as would hypnosis, but as local anaesthetic. One of the most vital concepts is that of the unity or the wholeness of the body. It is designed to restore the balance of the energies once again, and in the process restore the wholeness or the unity of the entire body.

Apart from using Acupuncture only as a means of anaesthesia and pain it is used as a therapy because it is suitable for treating a wide variety of diseases, ranging from internal medicine to women's and children's ailments, from neurology to organotherapy. It is often used in combination with modern medical processes. It generally takes effect very quickly, particularly in the alleviation of pain, and often proves more efficacious than chemotherapeutical preparations. It is a boon in malignant cases after surgery as a substitute to chemotherapy.

Acupuncture therapy has been combined with modern medical methods of treatment. Electric needles are also used (electro-acupuncture, galvano acupuncture). Veterinarians are having success in using acupuncture in the treatment of animals.

11. Magnetotherapy

Magnetotherapy is the system of treating patients through the use of magnets. Not only magnets but even magnetized water has been found to have very favourably acted upon human diseases and has worked as a beneficial medicine in many cases.

A magnet does not only attract iron but one of its healing properties is that it attracts all martial humors that are in the human system of blood, phlegm, black bile and yellow bile, of which the body in ancient medicine was thought to be composed. The magnet, therefore, is useful in internal and external diseases.

Magnetotherapy is both a science and an art. As science it is based on a natural force like electricity; as an art it involves the selection of magnets of different strengths to the different parts, to relieve different ailments of the body.

The treatment with magnets is not a new system, as with other therapies, like acupuncture, hypnotism, etc. The system was forgotten and became almost extinct for various reasons. But, it has been growing popular in the West though it is slow in development in India. This has led (as with other therapies and systems of medicine) to laymen practising without qualification and scientific background.

Magnetotherapy is used as complementary or supplementary to another system of medicine as and when needed. It has proved beneficial in certain diseases, especially in rheumatic and muscular aches and pains, as it has the power of draining pains out of the body.

There appears to be a close affinity between the principles of magnetotherapy and practice of acupuncture, acupressure, zone therapy. The trigger points could also be considered as 'magnetic points' for application of magnets on the human body.

12. Chiropractic

Chiropractic, spinal adjustment, is founded on the theory that vertebrae may become subluxated, that is, a slight displacement of their opposing articular surfaces may occur. As a consequence of this subluxation, there is produced an impingement upon the nerves which pass through the intervertebral foramen. This impingement is a direct result of the pressure produced by the altered position of the margins of the intervertebral foramen.

Ordinarily, when the word subluxation is mentioned, it is taken as disarticulation of the vertebrae but it is freely conceded that disarticulation of a vertebra is practically impossible without coincident fracture. Chiropractic, however, does not deal with luxation, but with subluxations.

As the spine is the central axis, or as it has been termed the line shaft of the body, every jar, fall, twist, jolt, to which the body is subjected, if it is excessive, can overcome the elasticity of the intervertebral discs and the tonicity of the ligaments, and it will produce a subluxation. The most common external causes of vertebral subluxations are, therefore, occupation, habits, injuries, age and exhaustion.

Subluxation is simply a slight change in the relative position of the contiguous vertebrae above and below it. There is not an absolute and entire separation of the articular processes of two vertebrae; on the contrary, the greater portion of their surface area still oppose each other; there may simply be a slight shifting of one vertebrae upon the other. This movement takes place in various directions, depending upon the configuration of the articular processes.

Were the vertebrae absolutely locked in position, even the slightest movement would be impossible, including even normal movement. But the fact that some movement between individual vertebrae is possible, is evidence that varying degrees of movement may take place, depending upon the force used to move.

The theory evolved is that when any part of the spine is dislocated, irrespective of the cause of the dislocation, the nerves leading from the backbone are trapped and prevented from transmitting the appropriate healthy signals from the brain to the organ involved and vice versa. As time passes the trapped nerve causes an irritation, poisons begin to accumulate and illness is the result. Subluxation of the vertebrae -- spinal lesion may be discovered by palpation of the spinal column and may be thus corrected by manipulation.

Hence the first principle of chiropractic -- namely that any interference with the nerve supply which has its source in the spinal cord and of course the brain, may affect any part of the body through the moving ramification of the nervous system. Next, the interference comes in the form of subluxation in the spine.

Where the abnormality in the spine exists or where the cause of the trouble exists in the spine, it is very probable that it will give rise to diseases and illnesses in any part of the body, however remote from the spine. Those are the very cases which need chiropractic treatment.

13. Osteopathy

The practice of osteopathy is a scientific adjustment by mechanical manipulations of the joints, muscles, tissues and viscera to promote the circulation and allow the vital fluids to circulate without interruption. It stipulates that disease is caused by abnormal changes in the tissues of ligaments, muscles and organs as well as in the position and mobility of the bones wherever situated in the body.

The practice of osteopathy is based upon a thorough knowledge of anatomy, physiology and hygiene.

Osteopathy differs from chiropractic in that it involves an examination and treatment of not only the vertebral column, but of every joint, bone, muscle and tissue in the whole body. It also slightly differs from chiropractic in the method of applying adjustment to the vertebrae, but as far as vertebral subluxations are concerned, they are identically the same for the purposes of osteopathy as for chiropractic. Also, palpation and diagnosis are made precisely in the same manner as in chiropractic.

Structural derangement is considered the most important underlying cause of disease -- what is called a 'lesion' may be in bony, muscular, ligamentous, fascial, or other tissue resulting in lack of normal movement in surrounding tissues allowing blood and lymph to stagnate, causing acidosis, irritating nerves which pass that way, and through them affecting the functions of various organs including blood vessels.

The theory evolved was that if there was a displacement of the spine -- the osteopathic lesion or subluxation, this would prevent the free flow of blood through the body, and the specific organs. If the life-force inside people, the blood, was impeded this would cause an alteration of functioning elsewhere, which in turn would cause disease or allow the body to become diseased.

Even constant physical stress can cause subluxation to develop and a whole series of anxiety states put together under the blanket term of nerves may develop and be wrongly treated as 'neurosis'.

Osteopathy premises that the body is a vital and physical mechanism, subject to derangement, structural alterations, and functional changes due to violence on the mechanical plane, as well as disturbances on the psychic and biochemic planes. Hence, osteopathic philosophy is inclusive of preventive, palliative and curative measures.

14. Differentiating between Chiropractic and Osteopathy

The main points of difference are manifest in the manner of application of the sciences, and the results of application.

The Chiropractor makes the spine the special and only locality of treatment essential to the cause of abnormal or disease conditions of all kinds. The chiropractic philosophy is defined as the adjustment of subluxated "vertebrae". The entire spinal column, is the field of battle as it were.

Whereas the philosophy of the science of Osteopathy consists of manipulations of the muscles, the adjustment of the bones reducing dislocations, removal of nerve pressure wherever found throughout the body for the purpose of freeing the circulation of the blood and other fluids of the body. In fact a general going-over on the entire body if found necessary.

While the object is the same, yet the means to the end are as different as if they have a different object in view.

It is advantageous to be familiar with both sciences so that much more good might be accomplished for the afflicted.

15. Hydrotherapy

Hydrotherapy -- greatest of all healing factors -- is the most beneficial system for human ills. Water is a great aid and powerful means of restoring normal functions in the body.

It is employed to help balance metabolism and in patients suffering from such disturbances remarkable results have been obtained. The latest researches and investigations carried out by the scientists have revealed the wonderful palliative and curative virtues of water. No other therapeutic agent possesses so many admirable qualities as does water. No other substance is capable of absorbing so much heat as does water, for which reason it is taken as a standard of specific heat. Being a universal solvent its use internally in the form of enema or colonic lavage or drinking water aids greatly in the elimination of waste products (auto-intoxication) which readily accumulate in the body under certain conditions causing more or less pronounced injury.

Hippocrates evidently had an excellent understanding of the physiological properties of water, both hot and cold, which he employed in the treatment of fevers, ulcers, hemorrhage, and a variety of maladies, both medical and surgical.

Other pioneers later built up a scientific hydrotherapy which is based upon definite and scientific data and is now recognized by eminent medical men as one of the most potent of all remedial agents. The science and art of hydrotherapy include not only applications of water in its various forms, but thermic applications made by means of hot or cold air, vapour and various heated objects, also heat and light.

Not all cases, of course, are curable, but even in those that are incurable, it is marvellous to note the wonderful degree to which pain and various other symptoms may be mitigated by accurately adopted hydropathic prescriptions. Water as a remedial agent is like potent drugs, a two-edged sword, and its unscientific use has not infrequently produced most untoward results.

Hydrotherapy is perhaps the oldest of all therapeutic methods, yet its versatility and its resources are so great by reason of the great number of variety of its procedures that there is always room for further progress.

Thermal Springs

Thermal springs, which have been utilised from time immemorial, have for centuries past been used to combat disease by effecting cures or for prevention. There are many varied chemical and mineral composition spas which provide a wide range of therapeutic treatment enabling each patient to benefit by the one appropriate to his specific complaint.

The waters owe their immediate and lasting efficiency to the presence, in active form, of one or more substances of recognized therapeutic value -- sulphur, carbon, phosphorus, magnesium, arsenic, iodine, calcium, copper, silicon, silenium, and such other gases as helium, argon and krypton. During the passage through the soil and the subsoil, the waters of the thermal sprays become charged with certain radioactive substances -- radium, thionum, actinium, polanium, and uranium -- and thus constantly bring up to the surface radioactive elements and rare gases which are diffused into the atmosphere. Hydro-mineral spas may thus be classified according to their therapeutic qualities. For long the treatment at the spas was one mainly of bathing and was conducted by empirical methods, but, during the last half-century the researches of scientists and the work of specialists have entirely revolutionized ideas concerning hydrotherapy. The specialization has been determined by scientific research on the physiological mechanism of their waters' 'therapeutic action'.

Valued as the waters are for drinking purposes, they are still more valuable administered as baths in suitable cases.

Besides the utmost advantage derived from thermal wealth, the spas have been provided with scientific and technical equipment which enable patients to benefit by the latest developments in medical science. The equipment for the administration of every form of baths is so complete that full advantage can be taken of the curative properties of the water.

Manipulation and massage in all its forms, are part of the cure. Immersion of the body in the water is an essential mode of treatment when radio-active waters are in use.

Now each spa specializes in the treatment of one particular group of ailments which may be of the following:

Affections of the respiratory tracts
Affections of the stomach and bowels
Liver complaints
Diabetes, gout and obesity, rheumatism
Affections of the bones and joints
Diseases of the heart, arteries and veins
Ailments involving the kidneys and urinary passages
Skin affections
Disorders of the nervous system
Disorders of the lymphatic system, anaemia
Women's complaints

Most of the spas abroad (unfortunately there are none in India) are equipped with material comfort, amusements, entertainments, and together with mental repose and peaceful environment take the patient's mind off his ailments and hasten his recovery.

16. Electricity in Medicine

The field of application of electricity in the healing art is a large one and the indication of its uses in therapeutics are plentiful. The effects produced by electricity may be classified as mechanical, chemical, thermic, actinic and psychic.

Pain and muscular weakness are the chief indications for the local application of electricity as a remedial agent. Another case in which it is most useful is that of neurasthenia and general nerve weakness. In certain skin affections and in some forms of malnutrition, electricity often produces good results. Its value in lowering high blood pressure is often remarkable.

By means of different electrical currents and modalities, we are able to cause powerful muscular contractions of voluntary and involuntary muscular fibres; stimulate the nerves and tune them to normal vibration, producing profound sensory effects; relieve pain or over-irritation and inflammatory conditions; dilate or constrict cutaneous blood vessels, and increase or stop hemorrhages; increase or decrease the blood pressure without producing heart depression; correct faulty metabolism, and hasten elimination of waste products, such as urea, uric acid, carbon dioxide, solidified lime deposits, etc.; harden or liquefy the tissue; produce anaesthesia and artificial respiration; decompose and introduce through the unbroken skin various remedies, direct to the seat of pain with a view to obtaining the desired effect.

Employing electricity in diagnosis, we are able to differentiate the forms of paralysis -- whether due to a brain lesion, or to lesion in the spinal cord - test muscular degeneration, locate foreign bodies, structural dislocations and malpositions within the body; differentiate various gynecological conditions, for example, pyosalpinx from ovarian neuralgia, etc.

In addition to the above-mentioned therapeutic properties, various electrical modalities have been found of special value in minor surgery, while the value of light, heat, ozone, and mechanical vibration produced electrically has been exemplified in the successful treatment of various nervous, rheumatic, respiratory, skin and other affections.

Sunlight is one of the greatest therapeutic agents known to mankind and, by exposing the body to its influence, many chronic diseases have been eradicated.

Actinotherapy, the actinic rays of the sun in concentrated form, is akin to sun rays. It has proved its great worth as a therapeutic agent in form of ultraviolet and infra-red rays used in hospitals and clinics.

Some of the future possibilities of electricity in therapeutics are the abstraction of metallic poisons from the body by ionization, safe local and general anaesthesia, with loss of consciousness and relaxation, relief of pain and the production of sleep, and so on.

Electrotherapy is not a cure-all, and will not take the place of all other methods, but it is a single remedial agent of a very wide range, leaving scarcely a condition of disease in which it cannot be used in some form, either as an adjunct or a remedy.

17. Remedial Massage

Man's original medical tool is his hand, which he has always instinctively used in order to alleviate pain. Whenever he is struck, stung, or seized with cramps, he involuntarily puts his hand to the painful spot in order to protect it or to rub, knead or massage it.

Massage is the methodical manipulation of the surfaces of the body by the hands of the operator. It is often combined with 'passive' and 'active' movements.

The effects of massage are manifold. It softens and relaxes hardened and congested parts. It forces out of the tissues the stagnant and impure blood, bringing a fresh supply ladened with oxygen and nourishment, thus ensuring rapid combustion and thorough elimination.

The beneficial effects of massage are exerted in different ways and for different purposes. Applied gently, it has a soporific effect (soothing action) upon the nerves of sensation, and applied more vigorously, certain methods have the effect of quickening the circulation of lymph and blood, and so leading to the rapid absorption of waste products in the muscles, and results in curing of diseases in various organs. Other forms of massage cause muscular contractions and so provide exercise for the muscles, in cases where movements of the whole body are not desired.

While it is apparent that one effect is to relax the muscles of the body, another is to improve circulation in which the poisons which are thrown up by the muscles much in the same manner as sponge soaks up water and then by squeezing discharges it. Other effects being to stimulate nerve activity, to increase lung activity, to quiet and soothe the nervous system, and to break up deposits in joints. There is still another mission or result of massage which is least understood and that is the transmission of vitality from the operator to the patient, as in laying-on of hands, which implies an energy flow from a healer to a patient.

In the premises of the foregoing, the masseur's (the operator's) object is to cultivate health, strength and personality himself. As he becomes more and more adept in his profession, his touch is more delicate but effective. A patient who has been administered a massage properly and scientifically in practically every instance feels immediately relieved of the symptoms of which he complained prior to the massage.

Generally speaking, massage increases the changes in the tissues and stimulates excretion thus increasing the bodily nutrition and activity known by the general name of 'metabolism'.

18. Exercise Therapy

Exercise sustains life. It occupies a unique position in relation to health. There may be any number of purposes in view with regard to exercise. Not only is exercise necessary for the maintenance of health and the building up of a shapely and capable body, it has also, in many instances, a specific curative value. Toning up the system will aid in the circulation of sluggish blood, with the objective of overcoming constipation. Defective posture, auto-intoxication and many other ills yield to a regime of exercises.

The two most important systems are physical culture and yogic *asanas*. Both are equally important, as the exercises employed ensure the harmonious development of the whole body and at the same time correct faults and deformities. A man's physical and mental education can hardly be considered complete without the introduction of some form of active recreation in the form of outdoor games.

Exercise and Rest

The first event of life is activity.

If any part of the body is allowed to remain idle it will rust. Therefore, use or lose; this applies to the brain and muscles, voluntary and involuntary parts alike. 'Life is movement, stagnation is death'.

All our activity, however, must have a definite purpose, and may be classified into four main groups: (i) productive labour (ii) recreative play (iii) exercise for development (iv) exercise for eliminating disease and regaining health.

Aside from dietetics, exercise is the most valuable therapeutic agent. Moderate exercise, both passive and active, will stimulate the natural function of all parts of the body and a craving for rest and recuperation soon manifests itself, as the rest condition is more often brought about by use of the muscles than by sleep.

Rest and sleep are not states of inactivity. They are states of activity, not necessarily conscious activity.

19. Fasting

Fasting, in the strict sense of the word, denotes complete abstention from food and drink but it is commonly applied also to the use of a diet somewhat severely limited either by the rejection of certain customary kind of food or by a diminution of the total quantity of food consumed.

Commonest by far, however, of all the users of voluntary fasting in the past and in the present time is its practice as an act of self-denial with definite religious intention. Fasting is practised for various reasons and a great diversity exists between mind and motives of men of different cultures and religions.

Apart from the most important preventive as well as curative measure in therapeutic fasting is its overhauling process and physiological rest it gives. There are three phases of metabolism: *Catabolism,* an overhauling process where water and tissues are discarded; *stabilisation* indicates that the eliminative process has come to an end, and *anabolism* is a constructive and a curative phase.

Fasting denotes abstention from food; while it is continued the body subsists on food material that has been stored in the liver and the muscles and accumulated fat.

The former are consumed first and then the store of fat. Later if the fasting is continued, the body will consume its own muscular tissue, but this is undesirable.

Fasting should not be carried out for more than three to five days except under expert supervision as acidosis can occur.

The fast should be broken very gradually; otherwise not only is the effect of fasting counteracted, but also danger to the system can be caused especially after a long fast. The bowels should be kept well regulated by means of enema or bowel wash.

The treatment is of considerable value in cases of indigestion, chronic intestinal toxemia and obesity.

Generally speaking, an occasional short fast for a day or two is advisable where there is a tendency to overeat and under-exercise.

20. Dietology

Dietology is altogether the most difficult of therapies, as well as the least investigated. It merits attention in proportion to its resources, from every practitioner. Not only that, but Materia Alimentaria should be the principal means of cure.

The failure of dietetics in certain cases is due to the folly of eating an excess of proteins, starches and fats and ingesting less positive mineral elements and vitamins.

The main purpose of wholesome food and a balanced diet is to provide the factors necessary for the growth and repair of the body and to provide those elements with which the body generates energy and heat. The two purposes strive for the maintenance of the vital force within us to the highest level of perfection.

Since body and mind are ultimately related, and ''you are what you eat,'' of all regulations for healthy living those pertaining to diet are the most voluminous. Of course food is not the only cause for the stability of the mental state, as the most healthful of foods, however, can result in the formation of diseases if they are not consumed with regard to the rules for eating.

In the selection of food we must take into consideration the taste, caste and creed as certain races have a natural affinity for a particular taste and can eat a particular type of food without suffering the ill-effects which may be expected. There are races which can consume hot spicy food without any thought for their pungency, whereas others would suffer from ill-effects.

The explanation for this phenomena in certain races is that hereditarily or genetically they get immune to the type of food due to their body's internal make-up.

It is desirable that no one should cook when in a state of indifference, agitation, sorrow and danger even though the person has the best of intentions for the fate of the eater, as the harmony is not likely to be optimal at this stage.

21. Rational Vegetarianism

There is another domain of natural science of vital importance to the welfare of humanity. It is the principal and practical application of rational vegetarianism.

Whatever one may think of vegetarianism as a continuous mode of living, a little consideration will make it apparent that a rational vegetarian diet is the *sine qua non* in the cure of so-called chronic diseases. In such cases every drop of blood and every cell is affected. In order to produce a cure the old tissues must be broken down and eliminated and new ones built up. The greater the change in food materials, especially if the latter are 'pure' and 'eliminating', the greater and faster will be the changes in blood and tissues. The same old poisoned food and drink will build the same old poisoned body. The less of morbid materials and the more of eliminating elements the daily dietary contains, the faster will proceed a complete regeneration of the organism. Anything short of this may be palliative but it is not worthy of the name Cure.

High cholesterol diets on health were clarified somewhat in the 1970s by explication of the effects of the two major types of cholesterol, high-density or alpha lipids, and low-density or beta lipids. The latter are health culprits because they can attach to the arterial wall, where they often build up in sufficient quantity to cause blockage of the type treated by bypass surgery. High density lipids, on the other hand, do not attach to arterial walls, but break down the beta lipids and help transport betas out of the body. Of interest is the discovery that strenuous exercise stimulates bodily production of alpha cholesterol. Many of the previous studies which had shown no correlation between heart disease and high-cholesterol diets could be interpreted in a new light. Some people, for example, had long been cited as a group with excellent cardiovascular health in spite of the enormous amount of cholesterol in their diet. A possible explanation for this might be that they walk miles and miles tending herds and in the nature of work.

Attempts to stimulate alpha production through medication or other artificial means is unwise, in that the long-term side-effects may be harmful and some subdivisions within the alphas appear to be as harmful as excessive betas. The best health strategy is to maintain a low overall cholesterol level through the choice of natural foods. Any effort to lower the beta proportion also should be made through food selection or through walks, jogging and exercises of the kind suited for the person.

Individuals who want to know their cholesterol levels should be aware that different laboratories use slightly different standards in their testing, so it is not possible to make automatic comparisons with published data, and it is best to stay with the same laboratory when keeping track of one's reading over a period of time.

With these considerations in mind, the decision whether to include dairy products in the diet becomes largely one of individual taste. As long as the entire fat content in the diet remains low, there is no observable harm in consuming some in the form of skimmed milk, cream, or fresh butter. Dairy products that have a low fat content can be treated like any other food, and the case histories of longevous people show that many used dairy products extensively throughout their long lives.

22. Colonic Therapy

The most despised and neglected portion of the body, the colon, has been found to be the most important organ of the body. The average colon in civilized communities is in a desperately deprived and dangerous condition. Nearly all chronic ailments especially of the heart, arteries and kidneys are the result of absorption of the poisons from the intestine, poison due to retention, constipation and delayed stool condition producing acute intoxication.

'Auto-intoxication', in medical parlance 'toxemia', means poisons in the blood. There is no subject in clinical medicine from which the condition of toxemia can be eliminated particularly as a productive cause or symptoms of all sorts. It may be safely said, therefore, that auto-intoxication is the underlying cause of practically all diseases to which the body is said to be heir.

Health is cleanliness. Cleanliness not only in the house, in the street, and in one's clothes, but above all within the human body. People who are meticulous about their personal cleanliness in every other way overlook one of the most important aspects of hygiene: the proper cleansing of the colon; that is why it is said that there is but one disease -- the deficient drainage.

Even though a person's bowels move daily, many are still constipated. Intestinal toxemia, rather intestinal sub-infection, is probably the biggest subject in medicine today because of the ill-effects and diseases it endangers. It takes into its range every organ and tissue of the human body.

A great many toxic conditions and in many instances, the primary focal area, have their origin in the intestinal tract, particularly in the colon which is overlooked.

The efficient treatment of colon stasis has always been a difficult problem. Catharsis, no matter how thorough, never cleans or disinfects the caecum. Mechanically the drainage is poor, and absorption of toxins into the portal circulation is responsible for much of the pathology in the upper right quadrant. Infection of the pelvis of the kidney by the colon bacillus is unquestionably blood-borne. The only possible cleansing and disinfecting caecum is actually to get into it.

Colonic therapy -- colonic irrigation, bowel wash or colonic lavage (one and the same) -- is a physiotherapeutic measure requiring just as much discrimination in application, just as much care and perhaps even more knowledge of human anatomy, as do other measures of physiotherapy which are deemed rightly the province of the physician -- and not of the lay-therapist.

Colonic therapy is by no means a panacea for all ills but deserves a great deal of attention because of the important diagnostic and therapeutic results that can be achieved through its employment. It is indispensable as a routine preparation for x-ray examinations of the gastro - intestinal tract, as one obtains a negative which is capable of much more intelligent interpretation if the bowel has been thoroughly cleansed of hardened fecal matter. It is also of the greatest value as pre-operative and post-operative treatment, bringing about improvement in the blood chemistry and hastening convalescence.

Physicians have found that drug therapy, different forms of electrical modalities, diet, may be used synergetically with this measure.

The universal effect upon human health of a diseased colon with its consequent absorption of the toxic products of catabolism into the general circulation, is recognized by many leading international authorities in all specialties of medicine and especially much emphasis is laid on auto-intoxication.

Colonic therapy is one of the most important therapeutic agents in chronic diseases especially in rheumatism, gout, arthritis, diabetes, heart, cancer. The chief object of colonic therapy is in assisting elimination of septic material from the body and restoring its normal function.

The main difference between an enema and a colonic is that an enema is a relieving process whereas a colonic is a corrective process.

23. Psychology

Mental Therapeutics : We have been dealing with the various arts of drugless science all of which involve mechanical and outward methods covering the physical aspects of human ailments. We now come to a totally different aspect of the care, the mental, the invisible where the only tools are in our own developed personality, will-power and magnetism. It involves the study of psychology as well as the physiology of the nervous system. It does not only take up mental effort and its products, but it includes habits, culture, behaviour, racial and religious customs, the lack of possession of will-power and finally the great problem of health.

Psychology may be defined as the science of individual experience, its condition, and its expression in behaviour. There are several schools of psychology in existence, each with a different set of principles and a different method of approach but in each the central problem is the nature of man as manifested in his various activities particularly those of thinking, willing and feeling, so far as they account for human conduct.

Applied psychology is the science, art and philosophy of thought action. The right mental attitude is of great importance.

There is an immutable law which says 'As within so without; cause effect.' In other words, the thought forces, the various mental states and emotions all have their effect upon the physical body. In any case, we must not lose sight of the mental influence on the physical, and equally the physical effect on the mental.

Throughout the ages attempts have been made to cure illness by mental therapy, but it is only in recent years that psychotherapy has been placed on a scientific basis.

The forms of psychotherapy used today are suggestion, hypnosis, psychoanalysis, and psychological analysis according to the principles of analytical psychology and individual psychology.

Hypnosis: Suggestion is the simplest form of therapy; a physician employs it whenever he assumes a bedside manner and whenever he assures a patient that his trouble is not serious and will soon pass. Its most potent form is hypnotism, the physician making strong suggestions. It is a method used to release the power of the mind by the introduction of a semi-sleeping relaxed state called trance.

Hypnosis has a great effect upon the human mind. It taps the subconscious mind, and especially, in cases of fear complex, inferiority complex, loss of confidence, mental aberrations, anxiety neurosis, examination fright, insomnia, stammering, obsessions, it has proved useful and effective in helping people.

It has now become a recognized tool of medicine, dentistry, obstetrics and psychiatry. It is extensively employed in obstetrics, gynaecology, paediatrics, psychotherapy and even surgery, as it is a perfect anaesthesia.

Hypnosis is the power of thought subconsciously working in a positive way which the mind has come to use when it needs outside help.

Hypnotism is a medical reality. It can be used as a powerful anaesthetic and as a tranquilizer. As a means of therapy, like another, hypnotism is considered an important method of healing especially in sleep, cure, relief of pain, obesity, psychosomatic troubles. It has become in effect a medical instrument but it is not an universal panacea.

Psycho-analysis: Psycho-analysis endeavours to trace out the root origin of the illness, and in this respect is more scientific than other therapeutic measures. The symptoms are regarded as a veiled language in which unconscious desires are finding a means of expression, and the aim of the treatment is to enable the patient to translate them into a more direct language, and thus to understand and control them. In doing this the patient acquires a deeper insight into the working of his mind and is able to overcome his internal inhibitions and correct any abnormal deviations. At the same time, he develops a measure of self-reliance and independence greater than that which he possessed before. The effect is thus the reverse of that achieved by suggestion treatment.

Individual Psychology: Individual psychology regards neurotic illness as a reaction against a sense of inferiority, a means of achieving a vivacious sense of power over one's intimates. Analysis, which is restricted to the conscious plane, aims at laying bare the way in which the patient has tried to overcome his feelings of inferiority and failing to do so has developed symptoms as compensations. In this way, it is claimed, the patient is induced to relinquish his strivings for socially useless power, and is re-educated along lines more in harmony with the life of the community.

According to Jung, the founder of the school of analytical psychology, every individual possesses four main functions by means of which he adapts himself to his surroundings - feeling, thinking, intuition and sensation. These are never equally developed in any one person; usually one function predominates, in which case its opposite becomes repressed. A neurosis arises when the individual is faced with a situation which calls for exercise of the repressed function; in other words, it is a conflict between the function by which adaptation is usually made and the opposite function, which through neglect, has been allowed to become unconscious. Treatment is directed toward enabling the patient to recover the submerged function, so that by a combination of the conscious attitude with the unconscious one a satisfactory adaptation may be made.

Psychosis: Strictly speaking, the term psychosis means a state of mind or a mental act, but it is generally used to denote certain forms of mental disorder which are to be distinguished from states of mental deficiency on the one hand and from the milder conditions of psycho-neuroses on the other. According to the latest classification the biogenetic psychoses are dementia praecox, paranoia, and the manic-depressive psychosis. Some authorities also include idiopathic epilepsy.

Like the psychoneurotics, the psychotics have their origin in an irregularity in psycho-sexual development, and are to be understood in the basis of fixation, regression, repression and consequent intrapsychical conflict. In psychosis, however, the fixation is in the very earliest years, or even months of childhood, and the conflict is between the ego and the outer world rather than between the ego and the unconscious. The chief difference between psycho-neurosis and psychosis, however, is the extent to which the repressed mental processes break through into consciousness after overcoming the resistance of the repressing forces. In neuroses the ego is unable entirely to repress the unconscious tendencies, but it can compel them to adopt a disguise before appearing in consciousness. These disguises in the form of symptoms represent a compromise between the two forces, the repressing and the repressed, both of which are equally active. In psychosis the ego appears to have given up all resistance and to be dominated entirely by unconscious mental processes. Its primary function, (that of subordinating satisfaction of the imagination to the evidence of sense perception), breaks down and there is consequently loss of orientation to the outer world. A new world is then created by the ego by means of hallucinations and delusions. In addition, all the later achievements of development, such as moral and aesthetic restrictions and inhibitions, disappear, so that psychosis may be regarded as a flight from reality, a flight from the adult form of existence back to that of early childhood or infancy, to a time when fantasy held sway unchecked by reality.

In a psychoneurotic, contact with reality remains unimpaired, and the repressed trends find expression merely as isolated symptoms like foreign bodies in otherwise healthy tissues. In a psychotic the barrier between the conscious and the unconscious disappears, and the unconscious dominates the whole personality. Psychosis has been aptly compared to a battlefield after all the soldiers on one side have been killed; neurosis to a battle still in progress.

24. The Missing Link

Instead of turning our attention to the cause or causes of disease, we keep pecking away at effects..

A great drawback in drugless healing is specialization in each branch of therapy. When patients resort to these methods, after trying various cures without success, they are confronted with different diagnosis.

If a patient were to step in an osteopathic clinic, he goes through a thorough osteopathic examination -- this is ''the Alpha and Omega'' of osteopathic wisdom and starts manipulating the joints.

The next one he consults is one who calls himself a 'Naprapath.' The Naprapath tries his best to discover any 'tightened' ligament which he thinks is liable to irritate nerves.

Then he goes to the 'Chiropractor'. He analyzes the spinal body, and all he cares to look for is ''majors'' and ''minors''.

Then he passes along to the 'Neuropath' who only looks for ''abnormal vaso-motor activity''.

Next he comes to the ''suggestive therapeutist'' who has a ''thorough'' knowledge of the ''power of mind over body'' and how to ''correct and harmonize mental influences''.

Then we have the 'Doctor of Biochemistry' who only looks for some ''deficiency'' of some inorganic salt in the body.

After going through all this, he perhaps ''slips in'' to the food scientist who claims that all ills are due to ''wrong eating'', and so he goes on through all the different methods of drugless healing.

Now who is right? -- What system will benefit him the most? -- and give him relief.

He does not care whether his trouble is due to slipped ligaments, subluxated vertebrae, lack of cell salts, or an abnormal mind.

He wants his health back.

Now who is it that is wrong?

Is it the Osteopath who only looks for mechanical faults. Is it the suggestive therapeutist who only looks for abnormalities of mind? Is it the food-scientist who only cares about the chemical composition of the body, or who is it?

Well, it can't be the Osteopath, because the Osteopaths have proved time and time again that disease can be caused by displaced ribs and viscera, slipped tendons, etc.

But is it not likewise true that the Chiropractor has proved that disease may be caused by spinal subluxations?

The Naprapath has proved without doubt that disease may be caused by contracted connective tissue, the Neuropath that disease is sometimes caused by disturbed vasomotor activity, the suggestive therapeutist that disease may be caused by an abnormal mind, the Doctor of Biochemistry that lack of a certain inorganic cell salt may cause disturbances, - and there we are.

Everybody is right. None is wrong.

As we have seen there are various therapies; so both practitioners and patients should not be carried away by taking to a particular therapy or a technique because it is in the limelight, or has become the latest fashion and a craze. Knowledge, understanding and caution on the part of practitioners as well as patients are very necessary as no system of medicine or therapy is a cure-all.

A practitioner should prescribe or employ a therapy or various methods as supplementary or complementary in a particular case, into his constitutional treatment bearing in mind that the proper selection or combination of the various drugless methods to suit a particular case is the main objective which a practitioner seeks to attain.

The popularity of alternative medicine is due to that it is only now that these methods are becoming more closely acquainted with the methods of a medical system based on scientific principles.

"Wisdom is a universal medicine, and the only remedy for ignorance, the great sickness of mankind."

This doctrine which some day must be the foundation of all enlightened therapy.

Part III

"Transgress the laws of Man, and you will spend your life in Jail -- transgress the laws of Nature and your existence will be a living hell."

-- Benedict Lust

25. Global Problems of Drug Abuse

The true extent of the drug problem shows an upward trend in the abuse of many substances, particularly alcohol, tobacco, nicotine, cannabis, cocaine, heroin and synthetic psycho-active substances, tranquilizers, and so on.

Drugs in themselves may not be the main problem as there is no such thing as a bad product. There are only bad users who have not learnt when to stop to save themselves from harm, which may even apply to many addictions like food, sex, religion. Their abuse is a profound problem particularly acute for individuals who are trying to cope with environmental stress. These drugs may become supporting crutches which in the long run are crutches that cripple giving rise to negative social and health consequences.

Those who experience a sense of inferiority, frustration, and other negative feelings, and thus gradually acquire a feeling of inadequacy and inability to solve their problems, reach breaking-point. When they resort to psychotropic drugs to relieve their anxiety these give them a feeling that they are living in a paradise on earth, not realizing that it will be a hell later as they become 'dependent' on these drugs.

Preventive approaches in the form of educational activities, not only for those who have not taken to drugs but also addicts who are motivated to remain drug-free after undergoing rehabilitation as the responsibilities with the individual, is not the final answer.

Take for instance alcohol addiction which is a major social and economic problem.

Alcoholics have always had a moral stigma attached to them and not considered a disease, because this definition is somewhat controversial as it is considered that no one gets to be an alcoholic unless he drinks.

There are a number of theories of addiction. Emotional upset theory: that people turn into drunkards in an effort to forget their troubles. This may be true for some people but there are quite a few social drinkers who have become alcoholics as well.

There are others who take to drugs or to drink not to escape reality. They do so in order to contact reality or inner reality feelings and an outer reality of human involvement.

There is also the ethnic or racial theory, that certain racial groups are more susceptible to alcoholism. This applies also to food, which is a matter of ethnic identity.

Whatever said and done alcohol is a depressant, narcotic, a drug and not a stimulant. It is an anesthetic, affecting first the high brain centres which control the voluntary behaviour and emotions. Alcohol is not a food. It can produce energy for the time being, it cannot participate in growth as it reduces the desire for food and drink; the utilization of food eaten results in nutritional deficiency diseases. There is a big difference between drinking and staying healthy, and drinking in order to get healthy. Drinking is something you can be healthy in spite of, not because of.

26. Stress

Anybody can keep going when the going is good.
Stress, the disease of the modern world, has turned
the main killer.

The stresses of life take infinitely varied forms and they can pose just as much of a hazard to health as bacteria, viruses, malnutrition or chemical and physical forces.

Insecurity, conflict in business or otherwise, family rows, dishonesty, commercialism, overcrowding and constricted accommodation, pollution, chaotic traffic conditions, noise pollution, frustration, loneliness in old age and lack of tenderness, surrounded by dangers, war threats, etc; all these syndromes and many more of the modern world bring about stress which causes more than any other single condition resulting in heart trouble, hypertension, cancer and even suicide and death.

Each man meets the challenge in his own way. Whatever the response, it involves the whole person, both body and mind play a part in dealing with the stresses of life.

The detrimental effect of too much as well as of too little stress is not so much attributable to external factors but rather to the organism's inability to cope with these factors.

A man reacts to his social environment as he perceives it, and the same environment may have diametrically opposite meaning to different people, even within the framework of the same general culture. For example, some men flourish on the freedom of retirement while for others it leads to a great strain causing what is known as 'retirement disease' which can even lead to an early death.

Indeed, physical causes of stress are now almost ignored as a result of stresses arising from modern society. The wide range of symptoms generally described as stress reactions are attributable to one basic and non-specific reaction. Once the vegetative nervous system has been activated a whole series of different physiological reactions are set in motion. Blood pressure rises, increased quantities of adrenalin are secreted, thus breaking down fat deposits and increasing the level of fatty acids and cholesterol in the blood. At the same time, the blood becomes more likely to clot and resistance to infection declines. Illness or infections following an initial stress reaction can thus arise in a variety of ways. A tendency of high blood pressure or heart trouble will accelerate. Reduced resistance to infections increases the body's susceptibility to infectious illness such as tuberculosis. The function of the gastric juices is disrupted, thus increasing the likelihood of gastric ulcer and even cancer, because the body when under stress, produces substances which suppresses the body's natural defences against disease.

It is said that man's "stress level" never falls to nil, if this was the case man would be extinct. As failure at times is a stepping stone to success or a trouble transferred into a triumph, so a certain amount of stress is vital for survival.

If too much stress is dangerous, lack of stimulation seems to be equally harmful. Some degree of stimulation -- both sensory and social is apparently essential to normal development, as well as to normal function.

It is only when the body is beset with an excess of external stimuli that stress can cause illness. To ascertain this danger level both the severity of the strain and the resistance of the individual must be taken into account.

The category 'psychosomatic disease' pertaining to any illness can be, therefore, influenced by what goes on in the mind, just as the state of mind is always influenced by what goes on in the body.

Throughout life there is a constant interplay between the body and mind and both require a certain amount of stimulation.

Apart from the conquest of health, we must also think of strengthening the mental, emotional and spiritual forces in us for the quality of life is more important than life itself.

As we cannot eradicate stress entirely, we must accept or try to learn to live with it physically, mentally and spiritually in the best manner possible.

27. The Toxic Society

Pollution is in the air we breathe, in the water we drink, in the food we eat. The nitrogen and sulphur oxides released into the atmosphere by various petro-chemical processes bring on an acid rain.

Lack of balance and deprivation of the humors in the soil are the main reasons for the present prevalence of such diseases and pests, and for the consequent increase of poison spraying with its risk to human health. The centre of toxicity is the industrial workplace.

It must be understood that cancer results when there is continuous insult to the body by noxious chemicals, as irrefutable research has established the link between cancer and work involving substances especially like asbestos-industrial dyes, uranium, glass fibers, and so on.

Risks from the air, however, are most serious in a metropolis where the industrial waste is trapped by skyscrapers and where automobile exhaust add to the toxic overload.

A dangerous escalation of environmental dangers is occurring with the introduction of nuclear power as a major energy source invoking the hazards of the possibility of explosion, the probability of accidents and the certainty of radioactive waste.

Perhaps the most underrated and misunderstood environmental pollution is noise, which usually is regarded more as a nuisance than as a health menace. While most recognize that impairment of hearing is a danger, it is found that excessive noise exposure is linked to cardiovascular disorder also.

Just as destruction is wrought by atomic bombs similarly many are affected by atomic force, produced in our own minds which generates the toxins in our bodies that kill us.

Intensifying all of these danger factors is the adulteration of the animal products now sold in the market-place, proved or suspected to be carcinogenous. A number of scientists, not linked to the government, have speculated that the soaring rate of breast cancer in women may be related to the different hormones routinely pumped into animals slated for human consumption.

To this health concern may be added the dangers posed by scores of antibiotics and other drugs that are known to have a negative effect on the human organism. Some are injected directly into the animal, and others are added to feed. Yet another hazard is posed by the many transmissible diseases carried by animals consumed by humans. The chance of infection is primarily guarded against by an antiquated and understaffed meat-inspection system which came into existence only after widespread abuses by meat-packers were publicized at the turn of the century.

Fish have fewer inherent drawbacks if they can be found in uncontaminated waters; but this is increasingly difficult, as many streams and lakes and parts of the ocean have become polluted through chemical leaching and dumping.

Chemical contamination of food reaches its zenith in its processed-and-packaged-food industries, where additives, artificial flavors, color, and preservatives are added. The overall purpose of these additives is to increase the product's profitability. The artificial flavor substitute for expensive natural flavor, the artificial color cosmetically disguises what has happened to the food during processing, and the preservatives extend the products' shelf or warehouse life. How successfully the body can handle these additives is a matter of bitter dispute.

Processed foods are so low on the nutritional scoreboard to begin with that the risks posed by additives make them totally unacceptable.

Additives, acknowledged to be toxic or carcinogenic, are common. Arguments bordering on criminal irresponsibility have been developed to the effect that the use of poisons in small quantities is harmless or an acceptable risk in view of the marketing advantages. However, different body chemistries have a different tolerance for a poison. So when it comes to individual use, there can be no foolproof safety threshold. Furthermore, chemicals interact when combined, so that taking in several different sets of additives in different foods, even if they are safe in isolation, can have unpredictable and possibly adverse chemical consequences.

Time and again, substances originally believed safe have proved to be extremely harmful.

Fresh fruits and vegetables are not automatically safe either. Although DDT and other dangerous pesticides once widely used are now banned, there are still more than five thousand approved pesticides, waxes, and colorings.

Fortunately, most pesticides, as claimed, do not penetrate the skin of plants, so thorough washing adds a considerable margin of safety. Even when a shopper is thrown back on produce grown by agri-business, the danger of consuming toxins is much less than with processed foods and meats. The least chemical contamination occurs at the lower end of the food chain. Thus root vegetables and grains have only fractional retention of pollutants, but meat, fish and poultry, all found at the opposite end, can have a high retention. Legumes, fruits and vegetables of all kinds also have relatively low retention. Dairy products are midway between the various meat and nonmeat categories.

Scientific discoveries reveal that certain vegetables store poisons when grown in poisonous soil and in turn poison those who eat them. Today poor health and diseases are due not so much to shortage of food as the lack of nutritional qualities in it.

One of the really difficult problems for the present generation is that much of our food no longer reaches us from the field, garden or orchard in the normal state as nature created it to meet man's nutritional needs. Such foods are now very largely collected and taken to large commercial centres, where they are altered, treated, processed, coloured, sulphurated, embalmed, adulterated, preserved, pickled, denatured, cooked, sterilised, pasteurized, and thus deprived of their vital elements. Whatever is left after being transported over long distances and stored indefinitely is sold to us in place of the original items which nature provided as food. Such denatured substances have no nutritional value but are junk being far from satisfactory substitute for natural food.

No form of life can be supported wholly upon laboratory products and man is no exception to this fundamental law.

Agricultural production is now undertaken mainly for commercial purposes. While agriculture may use commercial techniques to increase the production, the emphasis should first be laid on biology and then on technology.

Just as patients are restored to artificial health and to life with a drastic use of poisonous drugs causing depleted vitality or poor resistance falling prey to diseases, similarly modern agricultural methods by using sprays containing insecticides and pesticides for treating the soil, are confronted with the problems of plant diseases which are on the increase and which make matters worse.

Artificial fertilizers produce luxurious plant growth which is unbalanced and renders the plants themselves more liable to fungus disease and attacks by insects and other pests. A fertile soil is the first requisite to good health. The aspects of impoverished, depleted soil and the health of plants, animals and human beings should, therefore, be considered from the dietetic point of view.

The most drastic indication of the noncarnivorous nature of the human digestive system is its overall length and shape. The digestive tract of a carnivor is usually three times the length of its torso, as measured from mouth to anus. This shortness allows for quick processing and rapid evacuation so that meat does not decay within the intestine and give off toxins. The human tract is about twelve times the length of the torso, four times as long as that of the carnivor and one-fourth longer than that of most herbivores. The human system has a very long convoluted small intestine followed by a large smoother one.

Moral consideration aside, such an appraisal discloses that the high proportion of meat in the modern diet is inappropriate.

However, the mere fact that meat eating is gastronomically possible and generally convenient does not make it desirable, especially if meat is treated as a staple food.

A predominantly vegetarian diet with a high concentration of raw foods remains the best all-round bet for getting the proper essential materials.

Individual repose can reduce many environmental dangers but there is the danger of falling victim to some unsuspected source. The only acceptable permitted solution is general detoxication of society through control of pollution at its source; otherwise one has to suffer a planetary cancer epidemic or a global acidic rain.

28. Decision of Life and Death

The mystery of life is not a problem to be solved; it is a reality to be experienced.

Euthanasia is a Greek word and means "easy death". It is the deliberate termination of life.

Dysthanasia means difficult, painful unlimited death. Specifically, it is deliberate postponement of merciful death for days, weeks, sometimes years when everyone knows that the borrowed time will be spent only in misery.

It is true that life is an 'incurable' disease, that it must end in physical death.

The most acute world problem is whether to prolong life and suffering in the face of inevitable death. This is a very vital and debatable issue involving various problems--legal, medical, religious, moral and ethical--apart from a situation compounded with sentiment and emotion.

Let us endeavour to penetrate the essential pros and cons, so as to consider both its rightfulness and the profound difficulties involved in administering such a law honestly.

Had the patient, to be adjudicated for euthanasia, liquidation or killing, been competently cared for from the beginning of his illness that may have brought about the critical illness or injury? Is the extreme state of illness brought on by negligence, wrong treatment or by drastic measures through incorrect use or misuse of potent drugs, the side-effects of which are drug-induced iatrogenic illness?

The general medical opinion is that euthanasia should be permitted for those patients who are considered 'incurable', where there is nothing to offer by way of treatment. The main problem which arises in such cases is: who is to judge whether that particular patient is incurable, and should this be taken as the final verdict? It is a paradox when we find that many doctors say people are incurable when they are not. They have gone on living, despite professional prognostication of early death. No healing science is exact or perfect, nor are its practitioners infallible. Every science has its limitations, and so have the practititioners. Despite tremendous advances in the healing world there are limitations of a doctor in all fields of medicine. It is strange yet true that patients have 'miraculously' recovered when every rational hope has been given up. The question then arises: if so, how many such patients may there be? There may be very many, and they could be numbered only if there were enough co-operation from practitioners not only of one system of healing but of others as well. The practitioners of one system feel that theirs is the last word, which should not be challenged. Intolerance, bigotry and dogmatism are the greatest enemies of the healing art.

Let us be reminded of what a scientist had to say in this connection: "As a scientist with fifty years of study and research, I come to the conclusion that the things which we have said are impossible today become possible tomorrow, things we considered improbable today become probable tomorrow; and the cases considered incurable today by the professional men may be found to be curable by some other method tomorrow."

Isn't it factual, that the easy practice of legalised euthanasia undoubtedly would gradually reduce and retard the continued advancement of therapeutic research and scientific discovery provided of course the patient is not made a guinea pig for research?

But there is another side - the Agony and the Ecstasy

What drives people to take their own lives or take to self-annihilation or plead for death. It is not possible to understand them correctly and judge their motives, until and unless we appreciate what traumatic experiences men and women go through particularly before they take the extreme step.

Those clinically ill, sick of life, gone cases, dying by inches with humiliation, in coma for years, nobody or few to look after them, in poverty, a burden to the family, financially or otherwise. Such cases are not fighting against death but plead for euthanasia. "Mercy killing" a misnomer which should be "merciful death", relieves the terminally ill from the physical and mental agony, suffering and torture.

Even the patient's relatives mean this when they ask, "How much longer can this go on?"

Another most difficult problem one has to face is in the case of the aged and dying persons. Should their last days be unmercifully prolonged? When the death of an old, decrepit, demented 'vegetable' individual is inevitable is one justified in supplying 'extraordinary' or 'heroic' measures merely to sustain a spark of life? What about the emotional and financial strain then imposed for no good purpose on the patient's family? Does it mean really prolonging life or is it only prolonging the act of dying?

Many seem to think that the problem arises only of patients who are old, incurably ill and obviously dying but they feel the question of prolonging life is quite different when the patient is young or middle-aged. Distress usually arises in the problem of slow death when it comes to the aged whose race has been run.

Besides, what is the fate of children born with congenital malformations, physical and mental, who are a constant agony for the parents?

If a *Karma Yogi* wilfully discards his body embracing death for the liberation of the soul would he be stopped from doing so? Similar problem already confronting everyone is the distinction between euthanasia and dysthanasia.

There are zealous doctors who feel obliged to keep on fighting for the last faint heart flutter on the assumption that hope lingers for the patient until actual death.

The modern methods of resuscitation, it is said, would only renew the patient's suffering -- a miserable existence. Such attempted defiance of nature is even less justifiable than are efforts for prolonging life when the inevitable approach of death offers merciful release.

Hippocrates, the father of medicine, pledged physicians never to use a drug to produce death, but he also forbade the administration of remedies to those beyond hope.

Yet in both ways many seem duty-bound to do their utmost, keeping in mind that the dying might be allowed to depart in peace.

The opinion of late Pope Pius Xll is worth quoting: ''Euthanasia, deliberate provocation of death is obviously considered by moral laws. But with the consent of dying person, it is permissible to use narcotics with moderation to alleviate suffering, even if the narcotics hasten his death. In this case, death is not directly dismissed but is inevitable, and proportionate motives sanction measures which may hasten its advent.''

If euthanasia is made legal, with due respect to our healing profession, various problems are likely to arise, probably leading to misuse and abuse, including the tendency to cover-up instances of blundering, carelessness, incompetence, unskilfulness or even glaring crime in practice due to a sinister pact between the relatives of the patient and the unscrupulous physician.

Sir William Osler has said: 'Medicine is an art, not a trade; a calling, not a business; a calling in which your heart will be exercised equally with your head.'

If it is legalised, the law can be misused or abused knowing full well after all that there is no law which cannot be misused.

For instance the abuse of law in legalised abortion. Married or unmarried women, school, college, or working girls taking advantage of the law to cover up their misdeeds or guilt which is akin to taking of life as proved by the team of gynaecologists-cum-abortionists, who give up their lucrative practice as abortionists after watching the horrible reaction of the foetus during their experimental abortion, which they call 'the secret scream'. This is neither euthanasia nor dysthanasia but the abuse of law.

After going through the pros and cons, the rational approach seems to be that instead of generalising or making euthanasia compulsory, let there be a separate board or a panel of unconnected medical experts consisting of leading practitioners of different systems of medicine, knowledgeable in the particular field of medicine or surgery, and a member from the judiciary appointed by the Government to take the decision not mainly on the basis of what they consider 'incurable' but where it is found that the particular patient has reached a vegetative state having lost his mental faculties. Let it be prognosticated that even after recovery from his ailment, he would live in the same state. Then the patient may be adjudicated for euthanasia, with the consent of the patient, provided he is lucid enough to take the decision, or that of the closest relatives who will only act in the best interest of the patient to allow him to depart in peace and dignity.

This not only would help to scrutinize the case in question by the panel protecting the helpless from the risk of murder inspired by greed or other unethical motives, but it would also prevent the doctor, handling the case, to play God and act the judge to give the final verdict liquidating the patient *a la* euthanasia.

Besides, the method which may be adopted would not amount to 'killing' or 'murder' as by means of anesthetic the senses are deadened and with the increase of some lethal dose the patient to be adjudicated is put to rest purely on compassionate grounds with reverence for life. Just as people have a right to live in dignity, they should have a right to die with dignity.

Part IV

"Medical science has no frontiers, while every theory practised has its limitations; so a real practitioner will not say, "what is mine is good" but he would crave to learn and possess, "what is good is mine" in the interest of the patients and more so of himself."

29. The Art of Healing

There are two main schools of thought in the treatment of diseases, one is combative, the other preventive. The treatment of diseases depends on whether the disease is extrinsic or intrinsic, taking into account various other methods on the basis of analytical and synthetic viewpoints.

The combative method fights disease with disease-creating agents and the knife which suppresses the symptoms of disease, does not remove the underlying cause.

Medicine has been able to touch the exterior causes; when it comes to intrinsic causes it is another matter.

The extrinsic treatment of diseases mitigates the misery associated with the disease. It cannot alter the cause of the disease favourably.

The preventive method prevents it by eliminating the cause of disease by complying with the laws of health through health-building methods. Wrong living and the suppressive treatment of acute diseases creates chronic conditions.

The basic principle is that all healing comes from within the body itself, that is to say, there are self-curative forces which are inherent in the human body working towards health and healing. In reality Nature heals and cures, the physician lends intelligent assistance and interprets Nature's laws for the patient. *''Medicus Curat Naturae Sanat''* -- the doctor treats, nature heals.

Most people realize, however, that the body is self-curative where a cut or broken bone is concerned, but they fail to understand that this is also the case with disease as a whole.

The capacity of one organ or tissue to deputize for another has long been recognized. When a man has had the misfortune to lose a leg, his surviving limb grows so strong that after some time it is able to support the whole of his weight. When the valves of the heart have been so damaged by disease that they are unable to prevent a backflow of the circulating blood, the heart's muscle-walls compensate for the valve's insufficiency by thickening and pumping with such vigour that the circulation of the blood is maintained.

Health is the normal natural state of the human being, and it is maintained quite without conscious control by the wonderful, normalizing building, healing 'intelligence' which is sometimes called 'Nature' or 'vital force.' The inherent recuperative powers of the patient must be permitted to function freely and unhampered. It is that which heals wounds, repairs broken bones, builds blood, tissue and muscles, and eliminates waste matter.

In spite of the advancement of science and knowledge in the world of healing, sickness is very much on the increase. This is an inescapable fact notwithstanding the vast amount of money spent on medical research and the bringing into use of more and more 'wonder drugs' and sophisticated equipment. Too much specialization has led to reliance on technology, complicated as it is, especially being invested in diagnostic procedures of one kind or another as new tests keep being included year after year, more refinement in diagnostic power, but the outcome does not seem to help the actual understanding of the mechanism which underlies the disease in question. On the contrary the rat race of too much medical specialization has crept into surgery.

Despite the fact that medicine has progressed and there are on the surface wonderful successes with this or that particular ailment or malady, people complain constantly that the doctors are "too impersonal, too condensing, too busy to talk" and that on the whole there is a definite deterioration in physical well-being and increase in diseases like diabetes, heart trouble, high blood pressure, cancer and chronic ailments.

What we find is that the art of medicine is being overwhelmed by the science of medicine. A distinct division between basic science, and clinical medicine has been apparent. This approach leads to a deterioration of the physician-patient relationship. In fact, the progress of scientific medicine is felt by many to be outstripping the personal care of the patient to whom it is to be applied.

Medicine is not all science. Man has emotions and inner feelings which cannot be measured, although they profoundly influence his physical welfare. Bodily disturbances may be, and commonly are, the expression of his loves and hates, his passions and fears, his worries and anxieties; thumping heart, the cold sweat, blood pressure shooting high, and tremulous knees reflecting fright are but simple examples of this unity of body and mind.

Whither are we drifting? The question pertains not only to the field of healing but also to our mode of living. The parable of modern life is that it goes on fast but is reckless of direction, meaning or purpose; jet age living, injudicious eating and drinking habits, and so on.

The reason why most people suffer from various ailments and maladies is simply because they are ignorant of the laws of life. They fail to realize that they are working with a human machine. Often they do not want to know the facts, or are too sceptical or indifferent to investigate them; and those who do investigate and specialize in human machinery are trained to think and concentrate in terms of diseases and drugs only. Instead of emphasizing the values of personal hygiene, sanitation, the laws of health and stressing the right methods and principles of living by avoiding illness and maintaining good health, these specialists issue warnings against cancer, heart diseases and other ailments. This approach to health or disease is suicidal as it works very dangerously on the mass-mind, however intelligent it may be. Because of the miserable ignorance that asserts in matters of the body and mind people not only become disease-conscious, but the constant fear of approaching danger creates in them a psychological and emotional crisis ending in complete neuroses and pathological condition. There are curious instances of individuals succumbing to the very disease which they have most dreaded.

Besides our artificial civilization is encouraging evils destructive to sound principles. Custom and fashion are at war with nature. The principles enjoined and the indulgence fostered. are lessening physical and mental health, bringing upon the race an intolerable burden. Every person, therefore, must accept a certain amount of responsibility for his or her own recovery from disease or disability.

Lord Dawson, once physician to the royal family of England, said: 'What the patients want is a regimen and re-education in methods of living and treatments: it may be diet, physiotherapy and relaxation under controlled observation. Such treatment or education of the man and his tissues takes several weeks. We need a new type of institution distinct from hospital provision.'

We must not overlook the fact that preventive medicine enhances health more than the use of vaccines, sera and potent drugs for there is no better safeguard against diseases than good health itself. Positive health is the only true prophylactic or means of immunity against disease.

Immunity is largely a biochemical process where nature has endowed each species with a certain protective mechanism through which it can inactivate, destroy, eliminate, wall-off or otherwise negate those elements which would interfere with life and the normal functioning of the body. It is through these mechanisms that the body is made immune and is preserved against disease or poison.

Every illness no matter what its nature, is usually the consequence of a variety of causes, not just one, and no two people react to any one cause in the same way. The food he eats, the air he breathes, the genetic traits he was born with, the physical and mental stresses he endures, no less than the microbes to which he is exposed, all help to determine whether he will be healthy or sickly.

It is true that advances in health in the last century have been little short of revolutionary. Nevertheless disease of modern civilization is far from conquered, the fact that disease, we repeat, results from various causes such as environmental pollution, infectious illness, lack of hygiene and sanitation, the modern life-style, the physical and mental stresses of industrialisation and urbanization, the threat of radioactive fall-out and the hazards of exposure to noxious chemicals that are so freely discharged into our environment.

The stresses of life -- whatever the cause -- can pose just as much of a challenge to health as bacteria, viruses, malnutrition or chemical and physical forces. It involves the whole person, as both body and mind play a part in dealing with the stresses of life.

Incapacitated by one or more of the chronic diseases -- arthritis, heart disease, diabetes, cancer, the percentage of these illnesses has arisen alarmingly and there is a failure to respond to challenge. Even with increased bed space, hospitals are as crowded, in fact overcrowded, today.

Unfortunately, the almost total neglect of the laws of health and the universal use of drugs, sera, vaccines, antibiotics to cure disease produce a will-o'-the-wisp state of affairs. No sooner is one disease considered cured than a new one is born from it. This is fully recognized by the medical profession itself. To quote the British Medical Journals: ''As soon as we get an effective bactericidal agent, up crops the resistant strain, as soon as we immunize infants we get a susceptible adult population, as soon as we find the cause of a group disease and their specific treatment a new organism appears, e.g., the new virus still awaiting a viricide.''

Hence the civilized population are stripped of their natural immunities, leaving them acutely vulnerable when virulent germs do attack.

''Kill the germs and cure the disease'' is the watch-word of modern medical science. If you go germ-hunting for every disease that you have got or are going to get, there will be no end to inoculations, vaccinations, sera, and so on, poisoning the system in the belief that we are really immunizing the body 'scientifically'.

We should realize that in spite of the advances in technology and science one is not likely to succeed in wiping out the microbes that can cause disease. They are too prolific, too adaptable and too widespread to be made to disappear from the face of the earth. Nor can vaccines supply the whole answer. So many kinds of bacteria and viruses exist that at present it is impossible to vaccinate people against them.

To complicate matters further, some germs have an alarming way of developing new strains that are unaffected by existing vaccines and drugs as antibiotic use causes problems such as the microbes developing antibiotic-resistant strains.

Thanks to drugs of course man's burden of illness is generally eased whereas new drugs are manufactured almost every few months, then discarded, as offering nothing better than the old. This wild goose chase goes on while sickness and degeneration continue.

Prevention is the main weapon in combating disease. It is common knowledge that it is easier to prevent a disease than to effect a cure.

Among the rich death occurs owing to the disease of affluence while the poor owe it to lack of adequate health care, insanitary living conditions, non-availability of safe water and other causes. Both the rich and the poor alike die due to preventible causes.

Some time back the World Health Organization (WHO) adopted a global strategy aimed at achieving health for all by the year 2000 whereas we find that the art of healing has drifted further and further away from Nature. Basic issues like preventive medicine especially prevention of food adulteration, pollution, hygiene, sanitation, environmental hazards and natural and rational methods of healing are lost sight of.

It is too frequently forgotten, therefore, we repeat and emphasize, that the true art of medicine is not only to cure disease but to prevent it. The object of preventive medicine can be summarised as efforts to fortify the individual so that his capacity and powers of resistance are increased, to remove or prevent the causes of disease and thus to prolong the useful span of life.

So long as devastating drugs and injections are administered indiscriminately for immediate relief without realising their direct consequences -- the side-effects causing drug-induced iatrogenic illness which is worse than the disease -- and so long as the approach to ailments and diseases is by shot-gun, combative, symptomatic and suppressive measures, without removing or preventing the activating cause or causes of disease, and neglecting to treat the man as a whole, disease will be widespread. Unless there is a change from the so-called artificial civilized life-style to near normal and natural healthy life-style, new diseases of civilization -- degenerative and refractory diseases -- will not only increase but will remain a challenge, and health for all will be a mirage.

30. Conclusion

National Health a disgrace

There is hardly a person to whom the question of health is not a matter of interest and concern. The incidence of sickness is exceedingly high in this country, and a vast number of people live through a life-time of low and indifferent health. The consequent pain and suffering which innumerable individuals and families undergo defy description and the nation's loss, on this account, can hardly be measured.

In an industrial age in which we are living, it is not always possible to evade a stereotyped pattern of life which overlooks the importance of health acquisitiveness. But it is an indisputable fact that neglect of this faculty of ours brings in its trail ill-health, disease, suffering and premature death.

Yet the sufferings and the loss are not all inevitable. Much of this scourge can be avoided by widespread education of the people in the principles and methods of health maintenance and a general enlightenment of the public with regard to the lines and techniques of treatment which have yielded the best results in particular conditions and circumstances. For want of positive guidance based on scientific tests large numbers of people continue to grope in the darkness, flitting from one system of treatment to another, wasting their time and substance in a long and tortuous process of trial and error.

There is increasing recognition of the fact that vast scope exists for extending the reach of the healing art, and it is felt that steps in this direction should be taken with a sense of extreme urgency. It should be obvious that as long as a single human being remains without effective medical help, we must continue to explore new avenues of relief and cure. As long as a single malady remains without an appropriate remedy, we cannot afford to neglect any clue which might add to our knowledge of the secrets of health or the sources of disease.

Research may also reveal that various old and new substances and modes of administration have a range of curative or ameliorative action in relation to certain conditions, climes and temperaments and that diverse approaches to the problem of health and disease have complementary functions and are not mutually exclusive.

Various therapies and systems have made enough progress within the last century and a half to warrant us to utilize them to our best advantage.

Truth has many facets and error is a common human liability, and to the advancement of knowledge there are no limits. The plea is, therefore, that the door should remain open and the way made smooth for all earnest seekers of truth to explore widely and delve deep into the mysteries of the human system.

The complex of body, mind and spirit which constitutes the human being is indivisible until death, life cannot exist if one of these is absent. However, treatment of the individual can focus on one of these aspects, if the malady is more pronounced in one of them. The selection of the mode of treatment depends on a number of factors, the most important being the capabilities of the doctor.

Medicine must adopt a view of man as a whole recognising the unity of body, mind and spirit in successfully treating on the appropriate level as no total or lasting healing of the physical body can be achieved when the mental, emotional and spiritual elements have been untouched.

All said and done, whether a change of habit, environment, diet, it can prove valueless in enabling to map out the correct treatment of a case if we overlook the individual factor or what has been termed the 'personal equation' as each case must be treated on its own merits.

Commercialism and corruption in various forms have become so pervasive that the people have come to look upon it as a part of their moral existence and something from which there is no escape.

No physician should fail to recognise the merits of all branches of the healing arts. He should not attempt to make one branch of practice a 'cure-all' but should recognize the value of each therapy and a system when its need is indicated. The exaggeration of the benefits to be derived from any branch, method or modality is a positive way to hamper it and discredit his profession.

The patient's problem is paramount, no patient is a duplicate of another, therefore no standardized form of practice or technique can suffice.

Some remarkable personalities -- whose works will live for all times -- in the world of Healing: Hippocrates the father of medicine; Samuel Hahnemann in the field of Homoeopathy; Schussler in Biochemic system of medicines; Prieznitz, Lous Kuhne, Sebastian Kneipp, Dr. Henry Lindlahr, Dr. Benedict Lust and a host of others in the domain of nature cure; Sigmund Freud and his collaborators in psychiatry; Charaka and Susruta, who wrote the most well-known treatise on Ayurveda, Charaka on medicine and Susruta on surgery.

The great masters of the yoga system of health culture of ancient India, and others have rendered yeoman's service to humanity by their startling discoveries. They have revolutionized the practice of medicine and have helped usher in a new era in the preservation of health, prevention of disease and in the treatment of human ills of all varieties with their new healing arts.

It would be a matter of pity and great regret if we, who have had the opportunity to learn these healing arts from eminent masters and professors and have tested with positive results their superior efficacy on our patients, should remain silent and unresponsive to the call of human suffering and refrain from communicating these great truths to the world.

These observations and statements are not meant to prove the superiority or inferiority of any particular system nor are they intended to criticize any method.

The word 'integrated' is intended to emphasize its catholic approach and its multi-purpose character of the universal healing method. Health is the most prized of mortal possessions. The universal healing method includes all systems of right living and healing, a blessing for all mankind. The healing art is, therefore, man's greatest bequest to posterity.

The aim is to catalyze the serious investigation of alternative or unorthodox healing practice and its integration into a holistic system of health care in order to bring these vital findings to bear on actual theory and practice.

Hippocrates wrote on this subject: "Nothing should be omitted in art which interests the whole world, and which may be beneficial to suffering humanity and which does not risk human life and comfort."

Humanity is at the crossroads, not knowing which way to go. Bewildered and confused, not knowing what really constitutes the proper basis of life, mankind is heading for physical, mental and spiritual destruction.

Though it has long passed, it is high time those practising the science and art of medicine will reorient their thinking so that all branches of medicine get together and work with equal parity and in harmony for the promotion of health, prevention and cure of disease.

May the heartfelt conviction with which I have written this book, the message to suffering humanity, bear a rich harvest to my joy and to the benefit of my fellow creatures.

31. Humour Therapy
The Medicine of Mirth

A merry heart doeth good like a medicine.

Cheerfulness and hope are also important aids in maintaining bodily health and a sound mental condition. The bodily movements in laughter hasten the circulation and respiration and bring about general well-being.

The mental attitudes of patients have a lot to do with the cause of their disease.

Sir William Osler regarded laughter as the ''music of life''.

Mahatma Gandhi: ''If I had no sense of humour I would long ago have committed suicide.''

Abraham Lincoln: ''With the fearful strain that is on me night and day, if I didn't laugh, I should die.''

An excellent way to become a widow is to prepare rich highly spicy food, attractively served so that your husband would eat to his heart's content, then argue with him or nag him while he is eating.

A couple was advised to spend their honeymoon in the honeymoon hotel. They asked for a double bed. On the wife's side was written,

"I want you all the time". On the husband's side was a placard on the wall: "God give me strength."

Girdle: A device used to keep a woman smaller on the outside than she is on the inside.

Posted on the front of a jail entrance a sign that reads "amoeba" because it has only one cell.

Anatomy of Corruption: "All are naked in a bathroom."

Three Indians, while practising their English got around to discussing the wife of a friend who was childless.

"She is unbearable" said one.

"Arey Bhai, no that's the wrong word, She is inconceivable".

"No, no, no, no, you are both wrong," said the third, "what you mean is, She is impregnable."

A baby is one long alimental canal with a loud noise at one end and no responsibility at the other.

Dentist: The only man who can tell a woman to shut her mouth and get away with it.

Recipe for dating: Keep cool but don't freeze.

All tragedies are finished by death.
All comedies are ended by a marriage.

Poor Venus da Melo, imagine - a figure like that and no hands to defend her honour.

Vasco da Gama was the guy who circumcised the globe.

Temperamental: Ninety per cent temper and the rest mental.

It's usually a woman's geography that determines her history.

Padam's friend asked her to describe the first night of the honeymoon. "All night, it was just up and down, in and out, up and down, in and out. Our room was next to the lift."

"I finally cured my kid of biting his nails"
"Really, How did you do it?"
"I knocked his teeth out !!!"

Where are your bowels located?"
"I don't know. They move every day."

"Doctor, doctor, my hands won't stop shaking."
"Do you drink a lot?"
"No, I spill most of it."

The man believed so firmly in reincarnation that he made a will leaving everything to himself.

First Doctor: "Our patient is not dead yet. His pulse is quite vigorous."
Second Doctor: "No wonder; it is my pulse, you are feeling."

Jamsetji complained to his doctor
"I have this terrible problem. Everything I eat turns to gas.
I just had dhansaak and it has turned to gas."
"That could be serious," declared the doctor.
"But fortunately," Jamsetji went on "my gas is noiseless and odourless. Can you cure it?"
"I'm sure I'll be able to. But first, I'm going to fit you with a hearing aid and then I'm going to treat your nose."

When my friend's wife was in the hospital and was asked if she wanted a bed-pan, she replied "you mean I have to do my own cooking in bed?"

What is a traitor in politics?
A man who leaves our own party and joins the other side.

Then, what is the man called when he leaves the other side and joins our party?
A convert.

I was in my club the other day when I heard a man say, ''You know, Indian women are the best in the world. You just can't beat them.''
''Rubbish!'' snorted a companion, ''I beat mine everyday.''

''Look what I found in the Bible, Mum,'' cried Johnny excitedly running to his mother with a pressed dried leaf.
''Do you think it belonged to Adam?''

Before he gets married, a man yearns for a woman.
After he is wed, 'y' is silent.

Hysterectomy: An operation that removes the baby carriage, but leaves the play-pan in good condition.

''Daktar Saheb, my better half is suffering from lower half. I shall thank you from the bottom of my heart and my wife's bottom; please examine her inner space.''

Drugs, side effects, more drugs, more side-effects -- Doctor, couldn't I go back to the original arthritis?

''I want to know how long girls should be courted.''
''The same as short ones.''

An old man was mailing a Bible. As he handed in the parcel across the counter, the postal clerk asked, ''Anything breakable in it?''
''Only the Ten Commandments,'' he replied with a twinkle in his eye.

In the lounge of the British Parliament one young M.P. hesitantly told an elderly statesman that the fly of his trousers was open. While thanking the member, he quipped: ''Don't worry, young man, dead birds don't fall out of the nests.''

Said a young man: "Our oil stove exploded the other day, and it blew my aunt and her husband through the kitchen door into the backyard. It was the first time they had gone out together in 20 years."

"Any hope doctor?" asked the patient's wife.
"Depends on what you're hoping for," remarked the doctor quizzingly.

Marriage is like a pack of cards.
When you are courting its 'Hearts.'
When you are engaged its 'Diamonds.'
After marriage its 'Clubs.'
And at the end of it all its 'Spades.'

A clergyman and his wife were the chief guests at a graduation function of a women's polytechnic. As each girl came up to receive her diploma, she'd bow low to the clergyman. As one well-endowed graduate in a low-cut gown took her turn, the wife exclaimed under the breath, "By George, Did you ever see anything like that in your life Henry?"
With a straight face, the clergyman replied sotto voce, "Not since I was weaned."

A music critic noted for his biting comment was asked to appraise a promising sitarist.
"Immaculate," he observed and then added, "but no conception".

Marriage is an institution.
Marriage is Love.
Love is Blind.
Therefore, marriage is an institution for the Blind.

Meeting a minister on the street, his colleague said, 'you seem very happy to-day.'
'I am,' said the minister. 'I have given five adivasis great joy. I married two couples'.

'Two couples,' said the colleague. 'But that's only four people'.
'I know,' said the minister, 'the fifth was myself.'
Yes Minister, Garibi Hatao.

An Indian village housewife having got a job in U.K. tried to pick up the English language rather late in life but found it difficult to express herself.
After noticing with alarm the mounting totals of the grocer's bills, she wrote to him the following note, "Why are you so much dearer to me now than when we were first engaged."

The more we study, the more we know.
The more we know, the more we forget.
The more we forget, the less we know.
So, why study?

Don't do anything and after doing nothing, take complete rest.
That's Nature Cure.

FOCUS BOOKS

These books should normally be available at all good bookshops. In case of any difficulty in getting these books, they can be ordered from the Publisher. Please indicate the titles required and give your complete name and address including the Pincode.

You could order the books by V.P.P. in which case the current prices of books and the actual postage will be charged to you. Alternatively, you may enclose a bank draft or a cheque or a postal order payable to Popular Prakashan Pvt. Ltd. to cover the total price of books ordered and the books will be sent to you post free.

Every effort is made to ensure the accuracy of the price and availability of books but it is sometimes necessary to increase the prices and in these circumstances retail prices may be shown on the covers of books which may differ from the prices shown in this list or elsewhere. This list is not an offer to supply any book.

FOCUS ON HEALTH

Heart Attacks —
How to Recognise
How to Manage
by DR. NATOOBHAI J. SHAH
and DR SAILESH N. SHAH — Rs. 65.00

Are You Killing Yourself,
Mr. Executive?
by DR. R.H. DASTUR — Rs. 65.00

Sex Power
by DR. R.H. DASTUR — Rs. 70.00

Sex and Diseases
by DR. R.H. DASTUR — Rs. 48.00

What the Doctor says ...
by DR. R. H. DASTUR — Rs. 65.00

Stop Worrying about Backache
by DR. P.S. RAMANI — Rs. 30.00

How to Stop Stammering
and Start Living (2nd Ed.)
by DR. AJIT HARISINGHANI — Rs. 40.00

Full Life With Diabetes
by DR. A. S. GODBOLE AND
DR. A. A. GODBOLE — Rs. 70.00

FOCUS ON COOKERY

The Menu Book
by ANJANI NARAVNE — Rs. 65.00

Rasachandrika
by SARASWAT MAHILA SAMAJ — Rs. 75.00

FOCUS ON BUSINESS AND MANAGEMENT

In the Wonderland of Investment
by A.N. SHANBHAG — Rs. 95.00

Tax Planning for You and Me
by B.B. PALEKAR — Rs. 85.00

Understanding Business Data
Processing Systems
by ANUPAM BISWAS — Rs. 50.00

Professional Computer Programming
by ANUPAM BISWAS — Rs. 45.00

Computerising Your Business
by ANUPAM BISWAS — Rs. 40.00

How the West Grew Rich
by BIRDZELL & ROSENBERG — Rs. 60.00

GENERAL

The Last Days of Sardar Patel
(Original Filmscript)
by VIJAY TENDULKAR — Rs. 75.00

Crazy Bombay
by GANGADHAR GADGIL — Rs. 75.00

Rituals and Festivals of India
by TARA BAPAT — Rs. 50.00

Bhagwad Gita for You and Me
by M.S. PATWARDHAN — Rs. 50.00

Krishnarao Shankar Pandit
A Doyen of Khayal
by NEELA BHAGWAT — Rs. 50.00

Gita and Its Commentators
by S. H. JHABWALA — Rs. 65.00

Helpful Hints
by JYOTI SHENOY — Rs. 48.00

Krishnarao Shankar Pandit

A Doyen of Khayal

Neela Bhagwat

Khayal singing underwent a change in the eighteenth century, in both form and content, from the rigid and the mathematical to the romantic and at the same time divine. Loyalty and strict allegiance to the guru, in the authoritarian *guru-shishya* tradition resulted in romanticism being curbed. However, the early twentieth century saw the emergence of many other *gharanas* and with it developed many popular versions of *khayal* rendition.

One cannot assess the present without adequate recourse to the past. It is easier to comprehend and gauge and progress by intertwining it with the historical process and the aesthetic and sociological conditions which nurtured it.

This monograph, throws light on the *khayal* style of singing of one of the great vocalists of the Gwalior *gharana*—Krishnarao Shankar Pandit. Krishnarao was a towering personality of his age. Here is an attempt to understand Panditiji's personality and his contribution to *khayal* music in his own as well as the present socio-cultural context. The author has concentrated on the important themes in Pandiji's life—devotion to the father-guru, conflict with Pandit Vishnu Narayan Bhatkhande, career as a performing artiste. Guru and Principal of the Shankar Gandharva Vidyalaya and love for simple middle class life.

ISBN 81-7154-729-X

Rs. 50.00

FOCUS

FOCUS BOOKS
Division of
POPULAR PRAKASHAN PVT. LTD.
35-C, Pandit Madan Mohan Malaviya Marg
Tardeo, Bombay 400 034

Crazy Bombay

Gangadhar Gadgil

Illustrated by R. K. Laxman

Crazy Bombay brings together Gangadhar Gadgil's English writings, along with a couple of translations from Marathi, largely around the multi-faceted life of Bombayites. Some of these articles are autobiographical or pretend to be so. Gadgil has used humour to expose the hypocrisy and follies of contemporary life, sometimes as an interesting way of narration, occasionally for its therapeutic value and often to be playful, whimsical, boisterous or at times downright crazy and absurd.

Gangadhar Gadgil (*b.*1923) is one of the towering figures in Marathi literature. Known primarily as the standard-bearer of the new Marathi short story, his writings had an impact on the evolution of literary norms in the last five decades.

He has written over three hundred short stories, two novels, two plays, a number of one-act plays, several books of literary criticism. Yet behind this august output there is a mischievous mind, which has found free rein in his humorous writings in various literary forms both in Marathi and English.

Gangadhar Gadgil's English writings have appeared in the *Western Humanities Review, Illustrated Weekly of India, Mid-day* of Bombay, *Indian Literature* — published by Sahitya Akademi and *Triveni.*

ISBN 81-7154-719-2 **Rs. 75.00**

FOCUS

FOCUS BOOKS
Division of
POPULAR PRAKASHAN PVT. LTD.
35-C, Pandit Madan Mohan Malaviya Marg
Tardeo, Bombay 400 034